An Obstetrician/Gynecologist's Path

Amanda Malik • Michelle Iavicoli
Kahyun Yoon-Flannery
Editors

An Obstetrician/ Gynecologist's Path

What to Expect after an Ob/Gyn Residency

Springer

Editors
Amanda Malik
Department of Obstetrics and Gynecology
Cooper Medical School of Rowan
University and Cooper University
Health Care
Camden, NJ, USA

Michelle Iavicoli
Department of Obstetrics and Gynecology
Cooper Medical School of Rowan
University and Cooper University
Health Care
Camden, NJ, USA

Kahyun Yoon-Flannery
MD Anderson Cancer Center at Cooper
Cooper Medical School of Rowan
University and Cooper University
Health Care
Camden, NJ, USA

ISBN 978-3-031-87097-2 ISBN 978-3-031-87098-9 (eBook)
https://doi.org/10.1007/978-3-031-87098-9

This Springer imprint is published by the registered company Springer Nature Switzerland AG
The registered company address is: Gewerbestrasse 11, 6330 Cham, Switzerland

Preface

As you have probably realized by now, beginning a career in medicine is a series of ascending to the top of one ladder, only to quickly find yourself at the bottom of another. Through college, pre-medical coursework, medical school, and residency, you put in long hours studying, test taking, developing skills, and providing patient care. Graduating from residency (or fellowship) and starting an attending job is often the final ladder—although as you will soon find, there is no shortage of additional challenging rungs to ascend.

This book is one of a series, designed to provide newly minted attendings in various specialties with collective wisdom as to what comes next and how to navigate it. The field of obstetrics and gynecology is in many ways unique—part primary care, part surgery, part hospitalist medicine—and thus, you may find yourself facing unique challenges, especially throughout your early career. While we don't purport to have created a cheat sheet for every scenario you will face, we do hope you can come back to this book again and again, finding utility in the frameworks set forth by the authors.

When Kay and Michelle invited me to join them in this endeavor, it was easy to say yes—I felt like I was the target audience. Just shy of 1 year out of residency at the time, I had looked to my residency mentors and senior partners many times for advice and guidance on all sorts of topics, from the practical (where to find a job, what malpractice insurance to look for) to the more nebulous (how to guide a patient on a difficult decision, what next steps to consider for my career). We quickly began to compile a list of people we would want to hear from—some so familiar to me I could predict what they would write, and some so unknown that I wasn't even sure at first what chapter they might contribute. The diversity of authors and perspectives in this book is one of its strengths. While you may not identify with the words of each, you should find chapters that resonate with you.

For this reason, you will also find some overlap among chapters. The point here is not to be redundant but to offer you differing perspectives and include some nuance on the same or similar topics. In doing so, we hope you will find the tools required to reframe your own perspective when necessary.

Whether you stumbled across this book or got it as a gift, we hope you will find some useful wisdom in its pages. Though there are certainly valid frustrations with the modern practice of medicine and the field of obstetrics and gynecology, we also hope that this book will shed light into the passions and commitment of so many in our field. We—and you—are lucky to do what we do. Good luck!

Camden, NJ, USA Amanda Malik

Contents

Part II Your First Job Search

Part III After Starting Your First Job

Contributors

Lori Adriance Department of Obstetrics and Gynecology, Cooper Medical School of Rowan University and Cooper University Health Care, Camden, NJ, USA

Laura Brown Department of Obstetrics and Gynecology, Cooper Medical School of Rowan University and Cooper University Health Care, Camden, NJ, USA

Peter J. Chen Department of Obstetrics and Gynecology, Cooper Medical School of Rowan University and Cooper University Health Care, Camden, NJ, USA

Tyler Cholankeril Department of Obstetrics and Gynecology, Cooper Medical School of Rowan University and Cooper University Health Care, Camden, NJ, USA

John Chovanes Department of Surgery, Division of Trauma Care, Acute Care Surgery and Surgery Critical Care, Cooper Medical School of Rowan University and Cooper University Health Care, Camden, NJ, USA

Christina Chu Division of Gynecologic Oncology, MD Anderson Cancer Center at Cooper, Cooper Medical School of Rowan University and Cooper University Health Care, Camden, NJ, USA

Rori Dajao Department of Obstetrics and Gynecology, Cooper Medical School of Rowan University and Cooper University Health Care, Camden, NJ, USA

Meredith Crisp Duffy Division of Gynecologic Oncology, MD Anderson Cancer Center at Cooper, Cooper Medical School of Rowan University and Cooper University Health Care, Camden, NJ, USA

Richard Fischer Division of Maternal-Fetal Medicine, Department of Obstetrics and Gynecology, Cooper Medical School of Rowan University and Cooper University Health Care, Camden, NJ, USA

Jason M. Franasiak Reproductive Medicine Associates of New Jersey Lead Physician and Laboratory Director, Marlton, NJ, USA
Sidney Kimmel Medical College, Thomas Jefferson University, Philadelphia, PA, USA
Rutgers Robert Wood Johnson Medical School, New Brunswick, NJ, USA
Cooper Medical School of Rowan University, Camden, NJ, USA

Natali Franzblau Department of Obstetrics and Gynecology, Cooper Medical School of Rowan University and Cooper University Health Care, Camden, NJ, USA

Cosette Gabriel Contemporary Women's Care, Orlando, FL, USA
UCF Lake Nona Hospital, Orlando, FL, USA

Elizabeth A. Gagliardi Division of Gynecology, Lahey Hospital and Medical Center, Burlington, MA, USA
Department of Obstetrics, Gynecology and Reproductive Biology at Harvard Medical School, Boston, MA, USA

Allen Ghareeb Maternal Fetal Medicine, University of Washington, Seattle, WA, USA

Guy Hewlett Department of Obstetrics and Gynecology, Cooper Medical School of Rowan University and Cooper University Health Care, Camden, NJ, USA

Robert L. Hunter Department of Obstetrics and Gynecology at the Florida International University, Herbert Wertheim College of Medicine (FIU-HWCOM), Miami, FL, USA
Department of Obstetrics and Gynecology, Memorial Healthcare System, Hollywood, FL, USA
Acute Hospital Medicine, OB/GYN Hospitalist, TeamHealth, Knoxville, TN, USA

Michelle Iavicoli Department of Obstetrics and Gynecology, Cooper Medical School of Rowan University and Cooper University Health Care, Camden, NJ, USA

Neel S. Iyer David Geffen School of Medicine at UCLA, Section of Maternal-Fetal Medicine, Department of Obstetrics and Gynecology, Olive View UCLA Medical Center, Los Angeles, CA, USA

Joseph Maccarone Georgetown University, Washington, DC, USA
Cooper Medical School of Rowan University, Camden, NJ, USA

Stephanie L. Kass Northwell Health, New Hyde Park, NY, USA
Department of Obstetrics and Gynecology, North Shore University Hospital, Manhasset, NY, USA
Zucker School of Medicine, Uniondale, NY, USA

Shayan Khorsandi Pelvic Solution Institute, Vega Baja, Puerto Rico

Yon Sook Kim Department of Obstetrics and Gynecology, Cooper Medical School of Rowan University and Cooper University Health Care, Camden, NJ, USA

Kristen Knapp Department of Surgery, Division of Trauma Care, Acute Care Surgery and Surgery Critical Care, Cooper Medical School of Rowan University and Cooper University Health Care, Camden, NJ, USA

Kyle Le Reproductive Endocrinology and Infertility, Jones Institute at Old Dominion University, Norfolk, VA, USA
Department of Obstetrics and Gynecology, Cooper Medical School of Rowan University and Cooper University Health Care, Camden, NJ, USA

Lioudmila Lipetskaia Division of Urogynecology, Department of Obstetrics and Gynecology, Cooper Medical School of Rowan University and Cooper University Health Care, Camden, NJ, USA

Amanda Malik Department of Obstetrics and Gynecology, Cooper Medical School of Rowan University and Cooper University Health Care, Camden, NJ, USA

Saifuddin T. Mama Division of Urogynecology, Department of Obstetrics and Gynecology, Cooper Medical School of Rowan University and Cooper University Health Care, Camden, NJ, USA

Anthony Mazzarelli Cooper Medical School of Rowan University and Cooper University Health Care, Camden, NJ, USA

Jocelyn Mitchell-Williams Department of Obstetrics and Gynecology, Cooper Medical School of Rowan University and Cooper University Health Care, Camden, NJ, USA

Latisha Moreta NYC Health and Hospitals, Jacobi Medical Center, Bronx, NY, USA

Inara Omuso Obstetrics and Gynecology, MedStar Medical Group, Clinton, Southern Maryland, MD, USA

Anna Pancheshnikov Division of Urogynecology, Department of Obstetrics and Gynecology, Cooper Medical School of Rowan University and Cooper University Health Care, Camden, NJ, USA

Robin Perry Division of Maternal-Fetal Medicine, Department of Obstetrics and Gynecology, Cooper Medical School of Rowan University and Cooper University Health Care, Camden, NJ, USA

Karissa Rajagopal Department of Obstetrics and Gynecology, Cooper Medical School of Rowan University and Cooper University Health Care, Camden, NJ, USA

Carolyn Ross Department of Obstetrics and Gynecology, Cooper Medical School of Rowan University and Cooper University Health Care, Camden, NJ, USA

Michelle Salvatore Virtua Health, Marlton, NJ, USA

Alexander Santangelo Division of Research, Department of Obstetrics and Gynecology, Cooper University Health Care, Camden, NJ, USA

Kathleen Schaeffer Department of Obstetrics and Gynecology, Cooper Medical School of Rowan University and Cooper University Health Care, Camden, NJ, USA

Beth I. Schwartz Department of Obstetrics and Gynecology, Thomas Jefferson University, Philadelphia, PA, USA
Division of Adolescent Medicine and Pediatric Gynecology, Nemours Children's Health, Wilmington, DE, USA

Ciaran Smolinsky Department of Obstetrics and Gynecology, Lankenau Medical Center, Camden, NJ, USA

Lauren Spivack Department of Obstetrics and Gynecology, Rowan-Virtua School of Osteopathic Medicine, Stratford, NJ, USA

Simone Sweeney Department of Obstetrics and Gynecology, Cooper Medical School of Rowan University and Cooper University Health Care, Camden, NJ, USA

Carine-Ange Tagni SiBelle Med Spa, Women's Health and Aesthetic, Horsham, PA, USA

Stephen Trzeciak Cooper Medical School of Rowan University and Cooper University Health Care, Camden, NJ, USA

David Warshal Division of Gynecologic Oncology, MD Anderson Cancer Center at Cooper, Cooper Medical School of Rowan University and Cooper University Health Care, Camden, NJ, USA

Kristina Williams Department of Obstetrics and Gynecology, Cooper Medical School of Rowan University and Cooper University Health Care, Camden, NJ, USA

Laura Zalles Division of Reproductive Endocrinology and Infertility, University of Colorado, Boulder, CO, USA

Paul S. Zamostien Planned Parenthood Southeastern Pennsylvania, Philadelphia, PA, USA

Part I
Fellowships

Chapter 1
Applying to Fellowship

Stephanie L. Kass

Introduction

One of the major draws of OB/GYN is the broad and multifaceted nature of the field. Once in residency, though, or even before, you may find yourself particularly drawn to one specific aspect of the field. Those who pursue fellowship often want to narrow the scope of their career trajectory in order to become a more highly skilled expert. It can be daunting to think about continuing training for multiple years, but the investment in yourself and your career can be truly rewarding. You've already put in so much time and effort to get to this point—why stop now? This chapter will walk you through how to make this decision, considerations when doing so, and an overview of the process at large.

Types of Fellowships

At the time of this writing, there are six ACGME accredited subspecialty fellowships one can pursue after OB/GYN residency completion: Addiction Medicine, Complex Family Planning, Urogynecology and Reconstructive Pelvic Surgery (URPS), Gynecologic Oncology, Maternal-Fetal Medicine (MFM), and Reproductive Medicine and Infertility (REI) [1]. Additional fellowships that participate in the National Resident Match Program (NRMP) from OB/GYN include

S. L. Kass (✉)
Northwell Health, New Hyde Park, NY, USA

Department of Obstetrics and Gynecology, North Shore University Hospital, Manhasset, NY, USA

Zucker School of Medicine, Uniondale, NY, USA

A. Malik et al. (eds.), *An Obstetrician/Gynecologist's Path*,
https://doi.org/10.1007/978-3-031-87098-9_1

Pediatric and Adolescent Gynecology (PAGS) and Fellowship in Minimally Invasive Gynecology (FMIGS, or soon to be known as Complex Gynecology) [2]. Non-traditional fellowships include but are not limited to Medical Genetics and Genomics, OBGYN Hospitalist, Global Women's Health, OBGYN Quality and Safety, Women's Health Equity, Lower Anogenital Screening and Treatment, and Women's Imaging [3].

Decision Making

As evidenced by the breadth of options listed above, there are many routes you can take after graduation. So how do you decide? Think about what fills your cup during your day to day job duties. Is it the challenge of managing high risk pregnancies? The thrill of helping to create life? Allowing patients the freedom to make safe reproductive choices? Or is the operating room your true happy place? Whatever motivates you to feel most fulfilled during the challenging time that is residency is potentially something worth pursuing. Consider as well what you want your personal and professional life to look like after training and which career path will best align with those goals. Remember that choosing to pursue a fellowship means that you will be paid as a trainee for longer, but your income may be increased in the long run as a result. You are making a decision to delay some autonomy for the duration of fellowship, as your time is not your own in training, but that may result in greater autonomy in the future. Once you have decided to pursue subspecialization, and in which specific field, it is time to prepare.

Preparation

The early bird catches the worm. While you *can* match into fellowship with a last minute decision, your chances are much higher the sooner you start cultivating your professional life to achieve your goal. Start at your home program—does it have the type of fellowship in which you are interested or is there an attending who went through that subspecialty training? Find out what research they are working on and get involved! Ask for mentorship, and do not be afraid to share your goals. Get to know their connections—networking just may be one of the most influential things you can do. Attend whatever subspeciality-focused conferences you can and use that time to showcase yourself to as many people as possible by making a positive name for yourself! By carefully crafting your professional persona early on, you can set yourself up for a successful match.

Application Documents

Regardless of which fellowship you choose, most applications will require similar components: letters of recommendation, personal statement, USMLE score reports, CREOG scores, medical school transcript and diploma, curriculum vitae, and medical license/DEA. Make sure to keep a timeline and have necessary components well ahead of deadlines. Be strategic about who you ask for a letter of recommendation—consider how well they know you, their academic pedigree, and who they know. Make sure to ask early and be prepared to have to send gentle reminders. For your personal statement, really draw in the reader with an attention-grabbing first sentence and showcase yourself beyond the world of medicine. Give yourself time to acquire the documents needed from your medical school registrar as they are not always sent immediately. Double check your CV to confirm there are no errors. Don't forget to have a professional photo of yourself handy!

Preparing for Interviews

The nitty gritty on what to expect from interviews will be covered in the next chapter, but another aspect of this topic to consider is the process of preparation. First, let your administrative chiefs and program directors know you are applying in advance of the schedule creation. Depending on the type of fellowship, expected date ranges for interviews will be listed online. Give your schedule-makers this information so that you can possibly have a lighter monthly rotation, be able to coordinate with other applicants in your programs, and ensure that coverage is available at times of your inevitable absences. Find out if your program will allow you to take the day off to interview from home or if you are expected to virtually interview from your workplace, and if the latter, find a space that is quiet where you won't be disturbed. In the era of virtual interviewing, a good webcam and lighting truly may make a difference in how you are perceived. Be mindful of your co-workers, your environment, and your schedule in order to set yourself up for success!

Choosing a Program

Similar to the residency match process, the amount of control you actually have in determining your fate is limited. How important is the fellowship to you—are you willing to go anywhere to complete subspecialty training? Geography is important. Think about who else may be impacted by this big life change and make sure that they are included in your decision making process. Distance from family, ability for partner to be able to work, potential childcare difficulties, and overall support must be taken into consideration. Additionally, make sure that each program can get you to where you want to be by finding out where past graduates have ended up. It does not hurt to cast a wide net of applications and then narrow your list once you interview. During each interview, take notes in order to help you remember details when making your rank list. Only rank programs you are sure will be a good fit for your needs, as the NRMP Match is a binding contract. Ultimately, this will be your new living, learning, and working environment for the next couple of years!

References

1. ACGME. 2000–2024. Obstetrics and Gynecology. https://www.acgme.org/specialties/obstetrics-and-gynecology/overview. Accessed 20 Nov 2023.
2. NRMP. 2002–2024. Obstetrics & Gynecology Fellowship Match. https://www.nrmp.org/fellowship-applicants/participating-fellowships/obstetrics-gynecology-fellowship-match. Accessed 20 Nov 2023.
3. ACOG. 2024. Fellowship Opportunities. https://www.acog.org/education-and-events/creog/creog-clearinghouse/fellowship-opportunities. Accessed 20 Nov 2023.

Chapter 2
The Fellowship Interview

Allen Ghareeb

Section 1: Interview Process and Offers

Introduction

Prior to the COVID-19 pandemic, the fellowship interview often created a significant burden to the fourth year OBGYN resident. In addition to requesting time away from clinical duties, the interview process proved to be financially and physically taxing. The fellowship interview previously required two to three days of travel away from clinical duties, as the interview typically included a pre-interview dinner the evening prior to the interview. Hotel accommodations and travel arrangements were often left to the discretion (and the expense) of the applicant. The interview day typically began with an introduction to the program, followed by several interviews with division faculty, and often concluded with a tour of the clinical setting. One can appreciate the financial and time barriers this interview process entailed; it often limited the number of programs an applicant could apply to, and certainly the number of interviews an applicant could accept. The COVID-19 pandemic offered an opportunity to alter the traditional interview format and in turn, lower out of pocket costs to applicants. As the interview process became more equitable, more applicants could consider applying and interviewing at a larger volume of programs. Studies evaluating the impact of virtual interviewing on the match process have been overwhelmingly positive, with many applicants feeling that virtual interviewing provided them with the opportunity to consider cities they had never lived in or visited before and to rank programs in these cities higher [1]. As a result, the application process has also become more competitive. As access to fellowship

A. Ghareeb (✉)
Maternal Fetal Medicine, University of Washington, Seattle, WA, USA

A. Malik et al. (eds.), *An Obstetrician/Gynecologist's Path*,
https://doi.org/10.1007/978-3-031-87098-9_2

opportunities have become more equitable, applicants must become familiar with the nuances of virtual interviewing in order to differentiate themselves successfully.

The Interview Offer

In addition to changes in the interview process, many subspecialty fellowships have agreed to release all interview invites on a single day. While this day can be overwhelming and requires coordinated efforts at accepting and rejecting interview offers, it allows the trainee or applicant to map out the interview season well in-advance. Typically, interview offers are all released on the same day in late spring. Since moving to virtual interviews, the invites have typically been released the second or third week of May. While taking time away from work is not required to coordinate interviews, it is wise to sit down and have a calendar pulled up while accepting and declining interview offers. Many interview dates will overlap, and you will have to manage multiple time-zones. It is not uncommon to have multiple interviews in one day, in different time zones. Therefore, it is imperative that you are able to use a calendar to ensure interview offers that are accepted do not overlap. With the single interview invite day, applicants are not required to respond to interview invites in a "first come, first served" manner. Therefore, it is necessary to be diligent in understanding your capacity to interview in regards to time off from work, as well as the scheduling logistics required to complete interviews prior to accepting. Once interview invites have been accepted, you can begin to prepare.

Section 2: Preparation

Scheduling

If you are applying for a fellowship while you are still in training, it is imperative to ensure you have the protected time necessary to interview. While the virtual interview process has provided significant flexibility to completing interviews while minimizing time away from clinical duties, it is the applicant's responsibility to ensure his or her time to interview is protected. In order to do so, notifying program leadership and administrative chiefs of your desire to interview is of utmost importance. Secondly, once interview offers have been accepted, notify program leadership and scheduling coordinators right away so that coverage can be ensured. For many applicants, this will mean learning to juggle interviews from the hospital while briefly breaking from clinical duties. For example, at some programs, there is an expectation to complete clinical duties around the interview day (i.e., coming to round on patients prior to the interview or returning to clinical duties after the interview is complete), while at other institutions, there is protected time provided to residents seeking fellowship. Regardless of the program policies, it is the applicant's responsibility to ensure that interviews can be completed without interruption and without sacrificing clinical training time.

Program-Specific Preparation

As the saying goes, *you are interviewing the programs as much as they are interviewing you*. This is important to keep in mind, as fellowship is truly a unique time to decide what you want your specific skill sets and training to entail. For example, an applicant seeking training in Maternal Fetal Medicine may not desire to be solely focused on ultrasound and outpatient consultation and may desire more robust inpatient experience. Therefore, it is up to the applicant to ask the questions necessary to differentiate the training opportunities being offered by individual programs. Prior to your interview day, most programs provide you with an interview schedule consisting of various interviews with faculty within the division or department. Researching these faculty members prior to your interviews demonstrates genuine interest and preparation. Research the division to identify faculty members with similar clinical or research interests as yourself. If you find that there is a particular faculty member that you would like to talk to or shares your research or clinical interests and you have not been scheduled to interview with them, reach out to program leadership and inquire about the possibility of speaking to the faculty member during your interview day or at a later time. This will show genuine interest and enthusiasm to program administration. In addition to researching the faculty you will be interviewing with, spend some time researching the city in which the program is located. Questions to consider that often get overlooked but make a big difference in the day to day life of a fellow include:

- What is the cost of living in a particular city and is there appropriate compensation?
- Is public transportation readily accessible? If not, is parking covered by the institution?
- Is there meal money or stipends provided to fellowship trainees?
- If you are moving with a family, it is prudent to consider the cost of daycare or school, in addition to the feasibility of your partner moving with you and working remotely or finding a new job in the city. Is there support for partners of trainees?
- What is the average cost of a single-bedroom apartment for a single trainee?
- If a program is particularly far from family and friends, consider the accessibility of the airport and distance to travel.
- Consider your hobbies and activities of interest—are they readily available in a particular city?

Part of the fellowship interview process involves virtually meeting the current fellows. Typically, there is a pre-interview day social as there would have been prior to the transition to virtual interviewing; however, this has now been condensed to approximately an hour the evening prior to the interview. This is a great opportunity to learn about individual fellow perspectives and discuss the aforementioned questions. If you are not able to make the pre-interview, there is typically a portion of the interview day in which you get to meet with current fellows. This is also a great time to seek answers from the perspective of the trainee. Questions are largely centered on the location of the training program, as well the social community. This is a great time to assess how well the current fellows get along: *Do they spend time together outside of work? Do their relationships seem strained? Do they genuinely enjoy spending time with each other? What is the call schedule?* Some of these questions can be difficult to ascertain virtually; however, seeing fellows interact together generally gives the applicant a sufficient understanding of program dynamics.

An often overlooked part of the interview preparation is knowing your application and your accomplishments well-enough to answer any questions that may arise. If you have listed extra-curricular activities and research presentations, publications, or posters on your application, you should be prepared to answer questions about them. Questions can range from methodology of a particular research project to details about level of involvement. Failure to know your application thoroughly can result in being perceived as under-prepared or perhaps under-invested in accomplishments listed.

Location

Deciding on where to conduct the interview will likely vary by applicant. If you will be required to attend to clinical duties around your interview days, it is best to find a place in the hospital or clinic in which you can complete the interview uninterrupted. For example, many applicants complete interviews from a call room in the hospital. If you have the capability of completing interviews from home, there is more flexibility in deciding the appropriate location. More important than the location itself is establishing the key components to an appropriate setting.

1. *Appropriate lighting*: Ensure the location of the interview is well-lit and that your face is not shadowed in front of the camera. Placing your laptop in front of a window is a great way to use natural light to showcase yourself. If you are completing interviews from a dark room, such as many hospital call rooms, you may want to invest in a ring light as it will illuminate your face properly for the interview, even in the absence of natural lighting.
2. *Neutral background*: Find a calm and neutral backdrop to your interview. If completing the interview from the hospital, most hospital walls are neutral colors without significant wall decorations, but you should ensure your background is HIPAA compliant. When completing the interview from a private location or home, consider your background as a key component of the interview. Art or wall decorations can be used as conversation starters during the interview, but be

sure there is nothing displayed that you are not comfortable discussing. Be prepared to discuss any items that may be visible within your screen. It is best to double-check the interview environment before starting your interview!

3. *Quiet location*: It likely goes without mentioning, but ensuring the interview is completed in a quiet environment is essential. Whether that is from the call room at the hospital or in your bedroom, make an effort to minimize noise pollution as much as possible. Obviously, there are constraints, particularly to applicants who live in urban settings. If you have pets, ensure they are put away for the actual interviews. While pets are often welcomed during the pre-interview social hours, having them distract from your interview day can be regarded as unprofessional or may take up the relatively short time you have to make an impression.
4. *Desk*: Maintaining your camera at the appropriate height is important to maintaining "eye-contact" during the virtual interview. A laptop stand or textbooks can be used to elevate a laptop to eye-level. This also ensures proper posture during the interview and minimizes neck flexion over the camera during the interview.

Dress

The standard professional attire that has been expected for medical school and residency interviews is expected yet again for the fellowship interview. As the interviews are conducted virtually, often, the applicant is only visible waist-up to the interviewer. Therefore, many interviewees remain in more comfortable bottoms while maintaining professional attire waist-up. For those applicants juggling hospital duties and interviews, it is very possible that interview clothing is worn on top of scrubs; however, your outfit is a critical component of the interview. The best way to simulate an in-person interview is to dress for one. While trying to find the best interview outfit for yourself, consider that you do not want your clothing to distract from your messaging and your application. Therefore, neutral colors are often considered the most professional—but feel free to use color to express your personality—whether through accessories such as a tie or a colorful blouse. Jewelry that does not distract from the interview is also considered appropriate.

Once you have researched the programs you are interviewing with, prepared your background, and finalized your outfit—you are ready to interview!

During the Interview

One challenge with virtual interviews is that it is easy to become distracted; maintaining focus is more challenging when the interviewer is not in the same physical space. Therefore, you must be conscious to minimize distractions. This may include placing your phone in a separate room or out of your eyesight for the duration of the interview. You do not want to be caught distracted by your phone during the interview.

The more questions you ask during the interview, the more your interest in a program is portrayed. It is often best to have a set of questions that you can ask at each interview. Common questions include:

1. What research support is available to fellows?
2. Are there opportunities to apply for grant funding (i.e., WRHR, K-awards)?
3. Are fellows able to moonlight? If so, what are the restrictions?
4. Are fellows paid for faculty calls?
5. Are fellows part of GME unions?
6. Are there opportunities for home calls?
7. What faculty support is available on call?
8. Are there any anticipated changes to program leadership?
9. What are the program's biggest strengths and weaknesses?
10. Who makes the ideal fellow at your institution?

It is perfectly appropriate to take notes during the interview, and it is often encouraged, as these notes will help you when creating your rank list in the future. Take notes to remember how you feel on interview day and how your questions were answered.

After the Interview

Reflection

Taking a few minutes to reflect on the interview immediately after it has ended will serve you well when it comes time to make your rank list. A few notes on fellowship curriculum, research support, and how you interacted with current fellows will prove to be invaluable at the end of fellowship interviews. Notes do not have to be excessive; however, it is best to include details from the interview day that you can use in future correspondence with your interviewers. Writing a few words down about discussions had with various faculty can help demonstrate interest and gratitude to interviewers.

Post-interview Correspondence

Previously expected and customary, post-interview communication is no longer anticipated and at times discouraged. Make sure to pay attention to individual program requirements and preferences. Many programs will explicitly state that they do not expect nor anticipate any communication with applicants following the interview. If you are going to send thank you notes, ensure they are personalized and meaningful. If there are questions left unanswered from the interview day, it is encouraged to reach out to program leadership to ensure you have a complete understanding of the program. Many applicants will have different attitudes towards post-interview correspondence, with some applicants sending thank you notes to all interviewers, while some will reserve thank you notes and correspondence to programs of particular interest. Regardless of which strategy you choose, ensure that your communication is precise and meaningful. Many programs are limited in their ability to respond to such communication; therefore, it is important not to consider the lack of communication as a lack of interest, as there are strict Match rules regarding the amount and type of communication programs are allowed to have with applicants following the interview. Once you have completed your post-interview communication, your remaining priority is completing your rank list. Many applicants will consider sending a "letter of interest," or "love letter" to their first choice program. While certainly not expected nor required, it can show particular interest to a program. Programs may acknowledge receipt of such a letter; however, they are typically prohibited from responding to the applicant in a meaningful way. Therefore, response to a letter of interest should not alter the rank list. If you choose to send a letter of interest, make sure you only send it to one program: the program you intend on ranking first. It is considered unprofessional and disingenuous to send such a letter to multiple programs, as the Match can often expose such a discrepancy.

Conclusion

As medical education continues to adapt to the changes created during the COVID-19 pandemic, it seems that virtual interviewing is here to stay. As highlighted, the interview process has become more equitable and allowed for applicants to expand their programs of interest. However, as the applicant pool grows, it becomes increasingly more important for individuals to stand out during the interview. Through the tools mentioned in this chapter, applicants will be able to minimize the stress of interview planning and focus on their applications and themselves. The interview remains the highlight of the fellowship application process. Regardless of where you match, the interview is an opportunity to expand your professional network and meet potential mentors. It goes without saying, but remaining professional and cordial will serve you well for the Match and for career development.

Reference

1. Quinn KM, Runge LT, Parrado RH, Streck CJ, Abbott AM, Talley CL. General surgery applicants report the impact of virtual interviews on their rank list and match. Global Surg Educ. 2022;1(1):65. https://doi.org/10.1007/s44186-022-00071-8.

Chapter 3
The Fellowship Match: A Program Director's Perspective

Lioudmila Lipetskaia

When asked, "What are you looking for in a fellow?" I give an answer that is both truthful and unhelpful: "I am looking for a good fit for the program." This answer is universally truthful because all program directors (PDs) have a mission and are looking for team members who will help them execute that mission. However, it is unhelpful because it is not specific or concrete. There are many ways a person with different backgrounds and skill sets can fit into the program. Although there are some commonalities in how PDs choose their fellows, there is no single right way to demonstrate your value to the program. PDs are experienced and understand that shaping, morphing, and adjusting are part of the educational process. They are open to a variety of candidates but are ultimately limited by their environment and resources. They need to maintain and advance the program and look for people who can help them do so.

I am a urogynecologist by trade, and in this chapter, I will reflect on my process of selecting fellows for my fellowship. I could give you an ideal fellow description with a checklist of desired qualities. However, I do not think a mental image of a hard-working, responsive, always positive, extremely efficient, well-published, intellectually curious, emotionally mature, and socially capable team player will be helpful for you. Instead, we will look at the desired fellow features through the lens of the application process. Keep in mind, though, that this is ultimately a case report with a study where $N = 1$. It might not be directly transferable to every program director you encounter. I will try to highlight some common areas where I have validated my own experiences against my peer PDs, but at the end of the day, please treat it for what it is: an expert opinion, not an extensive qualitative study.

L. Lipetskaia (✉)
Division of Urogynecology, Department of Obstetrics and Gynecology, Cooper Medical School of Rowan University and Cooper University Health Care, Camden, NJ, USA

A. Malik et al. (eds.), *An Obstetrician/Gynecologist's Path*,
https://doi.org/10.1007/978-3-031-87098-9_3

We will start with your application. For the majority of applicants, this is your first opportunity to make a first impression. You will rarely interview only for the program where you are personally known unless you decide to go outside of the standard match process. Even if you favor the program where you did an outside rotation or were a resident yourself, you will have to write the common application.

There are common-sense mistakes not to make: do not leave fields blank, do not submit incomplete applications, and do not submit applications late. This will not necessarily eliminate you, but it will detract from your ranking score. Generally, these mistakes are seen as indicators of poor time management skills, sloppiness, or a lack of genuine interest in the process.

There are several important domains in the application: meaningful experiences, scholarly CV, personal statements, and letters of recommendation. I pay little to no attention to your medical school transcript, and I only care about your USMLE scores if they are extremely low.

When filling out the fields in the meaningful experiences section, include as many details as possible. Be specific to your work. There is a difference between: "I chaired a monthly wellness committee" and "While chairing a wellness committee, I established a support program that included twice-yearly, two-hour in-person education sessions on OR ergonomics and a peer-to-peer coaching program conducted bi-weekly. It was utilized by 50% of our residents and helped increase our engagement survey results." I am not interested in titles; I am interested in the quality of work you produce. You might not have a title, but if you can demonstrate through your application that you have established, spearheaded, and maintained something meaningful while doing busy clinical work, that will score you points. I am looking for the ability to achieve concrete results, and titles do not always reflect those skills. If your experiences resonate with my needs, I will highlight them on your application and ask for more details during the interview.

When compiling the scholarly CV portion of the application, highlight not only your publications and presentations but also your research skill set. I understand that your research output can be limited due to a lack of opportunities in your residency program. One publication from a community-based program will weigh more than three publications from a well-established academic residency with a large urogynecology division and multiple active research faculty. I understand that the time commitment, lack of mentorship, and busyness of clinical non-academic residency programs make doing research harder. Bringing it to the publication stage impresses me. This is also an opportunity to demonstrate that you are a motivated learner. Any statistics certificate you obtained or any collaborations and opportunities you designed for yourself demonstrate your resourcefulness and ability to elevate and advance yourself with little to no support. Research is important in any fellowship, and I appreciate research in any field, not necessarily in the field where my program focuses. If you have publications in gynecologic oncology or minimally invasive surgery, I do not treat it as disinterest in urogynecology when you apply to my field. The research skills are highly transferable, and it is the proficiency, interest, and drive that matter, not the field of application.

Regarding specialty-specific experience and surgical training, opinions may differ from mine. I, like everyone else, look closely at your OR performance. You need to graduate as a competent surgeon, and I need to know how good your foundation is so I can help you build upon it. There is no direct observation in the OR during the interview process, which would give me an idea of your strengths and weaknesses. I rely on your residency reputation in terms of surgical volume as a proxy for your skill set. I also look for independent observer recommendations. Letters from your home institution's faculty are somewhat helpful, but they are generally not specific or objective enough to highlight the whole picture. Fortunately, I have a very clinically heavy program, and even if you have limited OR exposure, I feel confident I can bring your level up as long as you have the right mindset. That might not be the case for every fellowship program, so to be competitive on their ranking list, you need to put evidence of your good surgical training on your application. Consider outside rotations, and when asking for letters, ask faculty to highlight your OR performance if you had a chance to shine during your outside rotation. This is as close to independent observation as it gets.

Letters of recommendation must be genuine and consistent. Generally, letters of recommendation are the biggest source of discontent for PDs. No letter writer is 100% objective as they are not evaluation letters but rather promotion letters. No letter writer uses standardized language to compare candidates' performance against their peers. PDs constantly need to "read between the lines." This is why it is preferred to have at least one letter from someone with a well-established reputation in the field you are applying to. I read letters from well-known faculty in the field and have a sense of how they vary from year to year depending on the candidate's strength. A good letter from someone well-known to me carries more weight than an excellent letter from someone I do not know. If you have no opportunity for an outside rotation, consider getting a letter from someone not directly vested in your fellowship match outcome. It is commonly perceived that your residency director or department chair wants you to succeed, introducing bias. An example of a less biased recommendation would be from someone outside your desired field or institution. If you are applying to urogynecology, a good letter from your gynecologic oncologist highlighting your surgical skills would be helpful. If they mention your interest in sacrocolpopexies during an eight-hour ovarian debulking case, it indicates that they were so impressed with you that they wrote a letter for a specialty they have no vested interest in.

Personal statements are my least and most favorite part of the application. I read them all and typically find one or two that truly touch me. Occasionally, I find quirky ones intended to stand out, and very occasionally, I find disturbing ones that are "red flags." These "red flag" statements are so self-centered that it is impossible to believe the candidate can care about anyone or anything else. A personal statement has never deterred me from inviting someone to an interview, but it does play a role in ranking.

In conclusion, your application is a portfolio of your "hard skills." Use it to demonstrate your capabilities and create an impression of your value. The next step is the interview process, which will test your "soft skills."

First piece of advice: Even in the modern world where interviews are conducted virtually, people pay attention to how you communicate. Any delays in responding to program coordinator emails, unreasonable last-minute requests for changes, or incomplete forms will leave a bad impression and will be noted.

The interview process is short and intense. I have limited time to spend with you and typically focus on your research interests. I rely on my faculty's opinions on other domains. Interviews, even virtual ones, are when candidates get the "vibe" of the program. This is when your enthusiasm, positive attitude, empathy, and personality come across. I make decisions based on first impressions, which can be inaccurate and prone to bias. This is why I talk to faculty and fellows afterward to confirm my impression against their opinions. It is always fascinating how one person on the interview team might have a completely different impression of a candidate. In such cases, we discuss and sometimes the argument is convincing and sometimes it is not. It is a team dynamic that ultimately tells me if we want this person on our team. Remember the "fit" idea we discussed in the beginning? This is where it becomes most apparent. We are looking for YOU to become part of US. There is no science to it—it is emotional, and it either feels right or it does not. You are also deciding if you like the program based on these interactions. This is how soft skills manifest—they make people want to work together.

Ultimately, I hope you understand that you cannot control the PD's perception of your fit. They know their program very well: its strengths, weaknesses, and needs at any given moment, which might change drastically from year to year. Trying to fit the needs of the PD is generally a poor strategy since there are too many nuances and not enough time to exchange information and get a full understanding. All you can do is present the best and most honest version of who you are and hope for a good match. Good luck!

Chapter 4
Gynecology-Oncology

Christina Chu

Introduction

Gynecologic Oncology Fellowship training has been formalized since 1973, first being accredited by the American Board of Obstetricians and Gynecologists (ABOG). Since 2017, with the transition of accreditation to the Accreditation Council for Graduate Medical Education (ACGME), the number of fellowships has grown from about 30 to 65, with existing fellowships now encompassing a spectrum from community to academic programs. Fellowships are 3–4 years in length, with at least 2 years of clinical training and, regardless of community or academic institution, at least 1 or 2 years of research. Programs can vary greatly in the volume and variety of clinical cases as well as the opportunities for research, so applicants need to carefully consider their interests and future career goals when choosing a fellowship. Due to the nature of the field, gynecologic oncology fellowship is considered the most rigorous of all the subspecialties of obstetrics and gynecology, and applicants should be well prepared to face the demands involved.

Application

Fellowships participate in the National Residency Matching Program (NRMP) and applicants apply through the Electronic Residency Application Service (ERAS). Generally, residents will apply in their 3rd year, with almost all programs adhering to a voluntary common submission deadline in April and issuing initial offers to

C. Chu (✉)
Division of Gynecologic Oncology, MD Anderson Cancer Center at Cooper, Cooper Medical School of Rowan University and Cooper University Health Care, Camden, NJ, USA

A. Malik et al. (eds.), *An Obstetrician/Gynecologist's Path*,
https://doi.org/10.1007/978-3-031-87098-9_4

interview on a date 2 weeks later. Interviews take place in the summer between June and August, with Match Day in September. Most programs will conduct online interviews with a few still using in person interviews. While the online process has advantages in cutting costs and eliminating some inequities for those unable to travel to many programs, unfortunately the electronic format may not allow applicants to get the full "feel" of a particular institution and its faculty and trainees. Many programs will host a separate online session with the current fellows to allow applicants the chance to interact in an informal setting without faculty present. Interviews are clearly an opportunity for the faculty to assess the applicant, but it should also be a time for applicants to gather as much information as they can about the program, including quality of life, as well as breadth and depth of experience.

The decision to apply to a gynecologic oncology fellowship should guide a resident's planning process starting as soon as possible. Demonstrating commitment and achievement in research is an important part of an applicant's portfolio. For many academic programs, this is an absolute requirement. Programs also evaluate scores of USMLE or COMPLEX, CREOG exams, letters of recommendation, and a personal statement. Applicants should take care to show commitment to the field of gynecologic oncology through their activities. Some residents who make the decision to pursue a fellowship late in their residency may wish to take a year after residency to pursue opportunities that may strengthen their application while they start the process at the end of their 4th year of residency.

A candidate should also strongly consider doing a one-month elective rotation at either MD Anderson Cancer Center in Houston, TX (a Rutledge Resident Rotation), or Memorial Sloan Kettering Cancer Center in New York, NY (the Brunschwig Rotation Resident Program). Both of these rotations provide second- and third-year residents an intensive clinical and academic experience in gynecologic oncology at two of the premiere institutions in the country. Residents will be assigned to a team and work in both the inpatient and outpatient settings. An elective rotation may be particularly important for residents in community programs or those that are less academic in nature. For residents from programs that have a lower volume of gynecologic oncology patients, these experiences can serve to give a potential applicant a better idea of what the field is really like before they commit to applying for fellowship. Both rotations will generate a standard composite recommendation that is well known and widely interpretable by faculty across the country. These rotations need to be planned well in advance and ideally completed in time for a letter of recommendation to be ready before fellowship applications are submitted.

Fellowship Experience

Most fellowships dedicate 1 year to research with occasional programs requiring 2 years. Applicants should consider what types of research are available. Some programs will expect the incoming fellow to step into a defined lab/project that has already been established. Other programs may have more freedom and resources to support a range of opportunities in both clinical and laboratory research. The types of acceptable research for thesis submission to ABOG are detailed later in this chapter and have expanded in recent years to include meta-analyses, quality improvement projects, mechanistic studies, and epidemiological studies, among others. Most programs will use the first year as the research year, which will allow the fellow to complete any remaining details and manuscript completion during their subsequent two clinical years, if necessary. In particular, those who are more interested in research or a future career in academia should try to assess the opportunities and support from the faculty for pursuing other concurrent projects throughout fellowship.

When it comes to clinical rotations, programs may vary greatly in structure. It is not uncommon for programs to incorporate one or more off service rotations on such services as the ICU, palliative care, bowel surgery, or radiation oncology. Regarding surgical experience, it is important to be aware of the number of cytoreductive surgeries and radical hysterectomies that are available to trainees. Applicants should also consider the balance between open, robotic, and laparoscopic procedures performed at a given institution. Some may be interested to ask about the fellows' exposure to bowel surgery, and whether the faculty perform their own bowel resections or if most exposure to these procedures is afforded on an off service rotation. The current procedural guidelines from the ACGME for programs are detailed in Table 4.1. Procedural minimums have not yet been established by the ACGME.

Consideration should also be given to how a program conducts training in the prescription and administration of chemotherapy and other systemic therapies. As the field of gynecologic oncology advances, we find that with HPV vaccination, the number of necessary radical hysterectomies may be decreasing, just as the radicality

Table 4.1 Gynecologic oncology procedural guidelines for programs with one fellow per year

Procedure	Number
Simple hysterectomy (vaginal, abdominal, laparoscopic, robotic)	75
Surgical treatment of cervical cancer (radical trachelectomy, abdominal radical hysterectomy, robotic radical hysterectomy, brachytherapy applicator placement)	10
Surgical treatment of ovarian cancer (Radical debulking, splenectomy, diaphragm stripping, liver resection, IP port placement)	40
Intestinal surgery (colostomy, bowel resection/reanastomosis, low rectal resection/reanastomosis)	20
Exenteration (anterior, posterior, and total)	2
Vulvar resection (simple, radical)	10
Vaginal resection (simple, radical)	no guideline set
Urinary diversions (continent conduit, ileal conduit)	2
Lymphadenectomy/sentinel node biopsies (inguinal, pelvic open laparoscopic robotic, para-aortic open laparoscopic robotic)	50
Number of cycles of chemotherapy (for each tumor site: cervical, ovary/fallopian tube, uterine, vaginal, vulvar, gestational trophoblastic disease)	100

of many ovarian cancer cytoreductive surgeries is decreasing as neoadjuvant chemotherapy is used more commonly. Rigorous training in the proper use of an ever expanding roster of systemic therapies is becoming more and more important to the practice of gynecologic oncology.

Research Thesis

An integral part of fellowship is the research component. By the conclusion of fellowship, an appropriate research thesis must be submitted to ABOG representing "significantly thoughtful and robust research effort." The prior publication of the thesis is not a guarantee of acceptance by the ABOG, and conversely, the thesis does not need to be published to be deemed acceptable. In general, the format of the thesis must conform to guidelines for an identified major peer-reviewed journal, must have a clearly stated hypothesis or purpose, and must represent work completed during the period of the fellowship. Reviews, book chapters, case reports, and case series (e.g., reports of the experience of a group of patients from a practice or department) are not appropriate. ABOG has expanded their acceptable theses to include:

- Laboratory, translational and animal research
- Randomized controlled trial
- Meta-analysis and systematic review
- Cost-effective analysis
- Case-control study
- Cohort study
- Survey research
- Epidemiology research
- Mechanistic trials
- Modeling and simulation-based research
- Quality improvement
- Qualitative research
- Artificial intelligence and machine learning research
- Implementation science

Board Certification

Fellowships have start dates of either July 1 or August 1. Given that the American Board of Obstetricians and Gynecologists (ABOG) specialty qualifying exams (AKA "obgyn written boards") are at the end of July, some fellows may prefer the August 1st start date to allow them to move to a new city and take their boards before starting. But the August 1st start date also means that fellows will be studying and taking their subspecialty qualifying exams (AKA "gyn onc written boards") during the last month of their fellowship, usually during a clinical rotation. Fellows with a July 1st date will be taking specialty qualifying exams during the first month of fellowship (for almost all programs, this will be at the start of the research year) and the subspecialty qualifying exams after completion of fellowship, allowing for more intense study during a time free of clinical obligations.

The ABOG subspecialty qualifying ("gyn onc written boards") and certifying (AKA "gyn onc oral boards") examinations will cover the non-operative and operative management for each of the major cancers (ovarian/fallopian tube/primary peritoneal, uterine, cervical, vulvar, vaginal cancer, and gestational trophoblastic disease), and where appropriate, the management of preinvasive disease as well. Complication of disease and treatment will be covered, including:

- Surgical complications
- Perioperative complications
- Complex inpatient care
- Radiation toxicities
- Systemic therapy toxicities
- Placenta accreta spectrum/obstetrical hemorrhage

In addition, applicants will be expected to understand post-treatment concepts including survivorship, surveillance, supportive, and end-of-life care. Topics relevant to the application of basic science to patient care will be covered including tumor biology, cancer pharmacology, pathology, radiation physics, and genetics.

Applicants should also be prepared to discuss the management of complex benign disease and the management of both surgical and medical complications. ABOG's blueprint for learning undergoes constant refinement.

After passing the qualifying exams, candidates may collect and submit cases to apply to take the certifying examinations which are conducted in person in Dallas, TX, at the ABOG testing center. It was a standard practice for the applicant to be examined on their submitted thesis as part of the qualifying exam, but with pandemic disruption of many fellowship research projects, ABOG decided to defer individual thesis examination for the time being. Applicants should be prepared to be examined on their thesis if ABOG decides to return to their usual practice in the future.

Mentorship

Throughout this process, the importance of mentorship cannot be overstated. Mentors are important throughout residency to help the resident shape their work and research to improve their application. Mentors in fellowship are also tremendously important to help guide learning and identify opportunities for excelling in particular areas of interest, whether that be in research, design of clinical trials, publication, or service on national committees. Mentorship and networking are also key in helping the successful fellowship graduation secure a job after training is complete.

References

1. *Gynecology Oncology Qualifying Exam—Blueprint and Bulletin,* American Board of Obstetrics & Gynecology. https://www.abog.org/docs/default-source/exam-blueprints/onc_2024_blueprint_updated_2024.10.16.pdf?Status=Master&sfvrsn=908d749d_3/
2. *Subspecialty Thesis Preparation Instructions*, American Board of Obstetrics & Gynecology. https://www.abog.org/subspecialty-certification/thesis-guidelines
3. *Subspecialty Procedural Volume Guidelines*, Review Committee for Obstetrics and Gynecology, Accreditation Council for Graduate Medical Education.. https://www.acgme.org/globalassets/pfassets/programresources/subspecialtyproceduralvolumeguidelines.pdf

Chapter 5
Maternal-Fetal Medicine

Neel S. Iyer

Introduction

Maternal-Fetal Medicine (MFM) fellowship trains Ob/Gyn subspecialists to manage complex obstetrical, medical, and surgical complications of pregnancy and their effects on both the mother and the fetus. MFM fellowships have been accredited since the 1970s. Currently, there are 95 programs with more than 130 fellowship positions, at both community and academic hospitals nationwide. Fellowships are typically three years in length, divided into two years of clinical training and at least one year of research training. There are a handful of programs that are combined MFM and medical genetics and genomics (MGG) fellowships that last four years and provide dual board certification upon completion. MFM programs can vary greatly in the volume and variety of clinical experiences as well as the exposure to both basic science and translational research opportunities, so applicants need to carefully consider their interests and future career goals when choosing a program. While MFM fellowship is not traditionally as rigorous as obstetrics and gynecology residency, it can be demanding, and applicants should be prepared for this as they decide to continue their medical training.

Application

As with all Accreditation Council for Graduate Medical Education (ACGME) accredited Ob/Gyn fellowships, MFM fellowships participate in the National Residency Matching Program (NRMP) and applicants apply through the Electronic

N. S. Iyer (✉)
David Geffen School of Medicine at UCLA, Section of Maternal-Fetal Medicine, Department of Obstetrics and Gynecology, Olive View UCLA Medical Center, Los Angeles, CA, USA

A. Malik et al. (eds.), *An Obstetrician/Gynecologist's Path*,
https://doi.org/10.1007/978-3-031-87098-9_5

Residency Application Service (ERAS). If applicants plan on starting fellowship at the conclusion of residency, they will typically apply in their third year of residency. Applicants can start their ERAS application in the late Fall with most programs having a submission deadline in late April. Interview offers are typically sent out in mid-May with interviews taking place in the summer between June and August. Applicants must submit their rank list by early September with Match Day typically occurring in the last week of September. Since the COVID-19 pandemic, most programs started and have continued to conduct their interviews online. The online process has significantly decreased the travel-related costs of applying to MFM fellowship. It has also decreased the time commitment required to attend interviews, often a constraint of a busy residency program. However, the lack of in-person interviews may prevent applicants from getting a full feel of the program and hospital. Many programs will often host an informal "meet and greet" with current fellows prior to the scheduled interviews. This allows applicants to interact casually with their potential future colleagues, without faculty being present. It also allows applicants to get a better feel for the "culture" of a program and ask questions that they may not feel comfortable asking faculty during their interview. While interviews are a time for programs to meet with and assess an applicant, they also provide the applicant with an opportunity to gather more information about the programs to which they are applying. Ultimately the applicant should find a fellowship program that aligns with their career goals and research interests.

The sooner a resident or potential applicant can identify their desire to apply to MFM fellowship, the sooner they can start tailoring their resume and clinical experiences towards becoming a successful applicant. Because research is a significant portion of the MFM fellowship experience, many programs want to see an applicant's commitment to research. While research experiences and publications do not have to be exclusively MFM related, they can provide a program insight into an applicant's research interests and desires for pursuing certain types of research as a fellow. Programs will also evaluate Council on Resident Education in Obstetrics and Gynecology (CREOG) exam scores, letters of recommendation, and the applicant's personal statement. Through their application, applicants should show their commitment to the field of Maternal-Fetal Medicine and their goals for fellowship and their career as a future MFM subspecialist.

If there is a specific program that a candidate is interested in, they should consider doing a one-month elective rotation at this program during the second or third year of residency, ideally prior to the application cycle in the Spring of third year. Elective rotations may be particularly important for residents in community programs or less academic programs, or those with less research experience. These experiences give residents a better feel for the fellowship and allow faculty an opportunity to get to know the resident better. This may give the resident a leg-up during the application process. If possible, residents should consider getting an additional letter of recommendation from faculty at the program where they do their elective rotation.

Fellowship Experience

All fellowships are required to have 18 months of core clinical MFM rotations and at least 12 months of research time. The additional six months vary by program and often include elective time, additional research time, or additional time on core clinical rotations. How this time, particularly the research time, is divided up varies by program. Some programs have established basic science research labs that they expect new fellows to step into for a predefined project, in which case the research time may be split into larger blocks of 3 months to a year. Most programs focus on clinical or translational research in which case the research time is typically split across the three years of fellowship. Particularly if an applicant is interested in basic science research, or if they are interested in a future career in research or academic medicine, they should note what research opportunities are available when evaluating potential programs.

The clinical core rotations consist of a minimum of three months of ultrasound, two months of outpatient MFM office, two months of genetics and genomics, two months on labor and delivery, and one month in an adult medical or surgical intensive care unit. Since one of the goals of MFM fellowship is to make a subspecialist competent in prenatal ultrasound and prenatal diagnosis, applicants should consider the level of hands on ultrasound experience that is available to them on these rotations, as well what portion of fellowship is dedicated to learning how to read prenatal ultrasounds. Similarly, if it is a goal of an applicant to remain actively involved in labor and delivery, they should assure they dedicate two months on labor and delivery. While inpatient antenatal care is not a specific core rotation requirement, most programs do include some inpatient experience. It is important to learn to care for critically ill patients in the inpatient setting and participate in procedures and surgeries, such as cesarean hysterectomies and abdominal and transvaginal cerclages.

Currently there are no procedure minimums for MFM fellowship; however, these will likely be established by the ACGME in the coming years. The ACGME does currently publish procedure guidelines for programs which are available online, and many programs have started to have fellows log procedures completed, similar to the case logging that is done in Ob/Gyn residency. Applicants should pay particular attention to the availability of the opportunity to perform and read fetal echocardiograms. While this is not a fellowship requirement, it is an important skill that can increase one's scope of practice as an MFM subspecialist. With the trend towards non-invasive prenatal screening (NIPS) and decreased emphasis on nuchal translucency measurements and serum analyte screening in the first trimester, the number of chorionic villus sampling (CVS) procedures has decreased nationwide. Applicants should inquire about hands on exposure to CVS. Most fellowship programs do not offer training in fetal therapeutic procedures, such as fetoscopic laser therapy or ex-utero intrapartum treatment (EXIT). Applicants may need to seek these experiences during their elective time or consider an additional fellowship in prenatal diagnosis and fetal therapy.

Research Thesis

As research is a substantial portion of fellowship, the research thesis is integral to completing fellowship. A thesis is required by all American Board of Obstetrics and Gynecology (ABOG)-certified subspecialties. It must be submitted to ABOG by the conclusion of fellowship and must be based on clinical or laboratory research performed during the fellowship period. The research must be important to the field of MFM and will be reviewed by the ABOG MFM subspecialty division for acceptability. Book chapters, case reports, or case series are not accepted to satisfy the thesis requirement. In recent years, ABOG has expanded the list of acceptable research for the thesis requirement to include laboratory or animal research, randomized controlled trials, meta-analysis and/or systematic reviews, cost-effective analyses, case-control studies, cohort studies, survey research, epidemiology research, mechanistic trials, modeling and simulation-based research, quality improvement, qualitative research, artificial intelligence and machine learning research, and implementation science. Each of these research categories has specific requirements that must be met to qualify for the thesis requirement, which are outlined in more detail on the ABOG website.

Board Certification

As with the ABOG specialty qualifying exam, the ABOG subspecialty qualifying exam for MFM is now offered annually at the end of July. The MFM subspecialty qualifying exam is a multiple choice exam that will cover medical complications of pregnancy, obstetrical complications, fetal complications and prenatal diagnosis, genetics and genomics, and core competencies and cross content. The specific content of the exam is outlined in the Blueprint for Maternal-Fetal Medicine and is updated on an annual basis. Each ACGME-accredited MFM fellowship should provide the vital clinical and educational experiences to successfully pass the exam, but potential fellows should plan to dedicate time at the end of their fellowship to study for the exam.

After passing the qualifying exam, candidates are eligible to take the ABOG subspecialty certifying exam for MFM. To take the certifying exam, candidates must already be board certified in general obstetrics and gynecology (i.e., taken and passed both the ABOG specialty qualifying and certifying exams). Like the ABOG specialty certifying exam for general obstetrics and gynecology, the subspecialty certifying exam for MFM requires applicants to collect a case list. The case list must consist of cases in three categories: medical complications of pregnancy, genetics/fetal disorders/fetal anomalies, and obstetrical and surgical complications. The MFM qualifying exam is offered every April at the ABOG testing center in Dallas, Texas. While a completed thesis submitted to ABOG is required to take the MFM qualifying exam, applicants are not tested on their submitted thesis during their oral examination.

Mentorship

Mentors play a key role throughout residency and fellowship to help individuals improve their skills and develop their interests and passions in the field. During the fellowship application process, mentors can be great resources to develop research interests, identify programs to apply to, discuss goals for fellowship, and plan long-term career goals. The MFM subspecialty world is small, and mentorship and networking are key to successfully completing Ob/Gyn residency, MFM fellowship, and at the completion of training when trying to secure a job. Potential applicants to MFM fellowship should consider attending national conferences. The Annual Society for Maternal-Fetal Medicine Pregnancy Meeting should be attended during the third year of residency. It affords a great opportunity to present research completed during residency and network in preparation for applying to fellowship.

Chapter 6
Reproductive Endocrinology and Infertility: Fellowship Applications, Interviews, and the Match Process

Jason M. Franasiak

Introduction

Reproductive endocrinology and infertility (REI) is one of the original officially recognized subspecialties in Obstetrics and Gynecology (OB/GYN) and among the earlier subspecialties in medicine. Recognized by the American Board of Obstetrics and Gynecology (ABOG) in 1972, fellowship programs are now 3 years in length following an OB/GYN residency [1]. Originally focused entirely on endocrine problems related to reproductive function, the assisted reproductive technologies (ART) have recently become the larger part of training during REI fellowships.

Embarking on a career in Obstetrics and Gynecology (OB/GYN) opens the door to a vast array of possibilities within the field. For OB/GYN residents who have developed a keen interest in REI, pursuing a fellowship in this subspecialty is an exciting prospect. In this chapter, we delve into the aspects of the fellowship application process, fellowship interviews, and the fellowship match process for REI.

J. M. Franasiak (✉)
Reproductive Medicine Associates of New Jersey Lead Physician and Laboratory Director, Marlton, NJ, USA

Sidney Kimmel Medical College, Thomas Jefferson University, Philadelphia, PA, USA

Rutgers Robert Wood Johnson Medical School, New Brunswick, NJ, USA

Cooper Medical School of Rowan University, Camden, NJ, USA

A. Malik et al. (eds.), *An Obstetrician/Gynecologist's Path*,
https://doi.org/10.1007/978-3-031-87098-9_6

Exploring the Field of Reproductive Endocrinology and Infertility

REI encompasses the management of various conditions related to fertility, hormonal regulation, menstrual disorders, and reproductive health. By employing specialized diagnostic tools and evidence-based interventions, reproductive endocrinologists play a crucial role in helping individuals and couples achieve their reproductive goals while addressing underlying health concerns.

In recent years, REI has witnessed remarkable advancements. ART, including IVF, preimplantation genetic testing, and cryopreservation techniques, have revolutionized the treatment of infertility. Additionally, the field continues to explore cutting-edge research in areas such as reproductive genetics, fertility preservation, minimally invasive surgical techniques, and personalized approaches to reproductive healthcare.

REI fellowships were originally 2-year programs. Today, fellowship programs have increased to 3 years in duration and fellow training encompasses reproductive surgery, ART including IVF and embryology, clinical training, reproductive science research, and didactic education, including biostatistics and epidemiology [1]. The requirements and criteria for training in REI are determined by ABOG. After satisfactory completion of an accredited fellowship, graduates must sit for the written exam in the subspecialty. Candidates who pass the written REI examination and have been certified by the general OB/GYN specialty boards are eligible to apply for the REI oral subspecialty exam. Once certified, specialists must complete ABOG's annual maintenance of certification (MOC) to retain certification status.

Preparing to Apply to a Reproductive Endocrinology Fellowship

Preparing for a fellowship in REI requires planning, engagement, and a strong application. OB/GYN residency is a busy time; however, engaging in research projects related to reproductive medicine during your residency can significantly enhance your fellowship application. Actively participate in ongoing research within your institution or collaborate with other researchers. Seek opportunities to contribute to publications, abstracts, or presentations related to REI. Research experience demonstrates your commitment to advancing knowledge in the field and showcases your ability to contribute to scholarly activities during the fellowship.

Seed out opportunities to attend conferences, workshops, and seminars focused on REI to expand your knowledge, network with experts in the field, and stay updated on the latest advancements. Consider presenting your research findings or case studies at relevant conferences to gain visibility and contribute to the academic community. Actively engage with professional organizations and REIs through networking events or mentorship programs, fostering connections that may strengthen your application.

A well-crafted curriculum vitae (CV) is crucial for an application which showcases your accomplishments, experiences, and qualifications. It should highlight your academic achievements, honors, research experience, publications, and presentations related to reproductive medicine. This can include your clinical rotations, participation in conferences, leadership roles, and any specialized training or certifications. You ought to tailor your CV and application to highlight relevant experiences and emphasize your dedication to REI.

Your personal statement is an opportunity to express your passion for REI and articulate your career goals. You should use this portion of the application as a way to convey how your experiences have shaped your interest in the field and demonstrate your commitment to advancing reproductive healthcare. Discuss specific areas of REI that intrigue you and mention any research or clinical experiences that influenced your decision to pursue this fellowship.

Choosing the right individuals to write your letters of recommendation is crucial. Seek out faculty members who have worked closely with you and can speak to your clinical abilities, research potential, work ethic, and dedication to reproductive medicine. Reach out to potential recommenders well in advance, providing them with relevant information about your goals, experiences, and a deadline for submission. Remember to follow up and express your gratitude once the letters have been submitted.

Finally, you should thoroughly research fellowship programs to identify those that align with your career goals and offer the training and resources you seek. Explore program websites and review their faculty profiles, publications, and ongoing research. Consider factors such as program reputation, clinical exposure, research opportunities, mentoring, geographic location, and the track record of previous fellows.

The Fellowship Application Process

According to the Society of Reproductive Endocrinology and Infertility, there are 49 fellowship programs in REI for the 2023–2024 academic year [2]. The application process utilizes the Electronic Residency Application Service (ERAS) system and applications are typically due in May of the application year. Create an account, gather the necessary documentation, and follow the platform's instructions for submitting your application materials electronically. Mark important dates on your calendar to ensure you submit your application materials on time.

Carefully review the specific application requirements of each fellowship program. Common documents include your curriculum vitae (CV), personal statement, academic transcripts, letters of recommendation, and USMLE scores. Some programs may also require additional documents such as a list of completed rotations, a photograph, or a cover letter. Ensure that all required documents are properly formatted, accurately represent your achievements, and meet the program's guidelines.

Each fellowship program may have unique requirements or preferences. Some programs may prioritize candidates with specific research interests, clinical experiences, or prior exposure to certain procedures. Research each program's website and contact their program coordinator or director if you have any questions about their specific expectations.

Pay close attention to detail to ensure your application is complete and error-free. Proofread all written components, including your personal statement, for grammar, spelling, and content accuracy. Ask trusted colleagues or mentors to review your application materials for feedback and suggestions. Ensure that all supporting documents, such as transcripts and letters of recommendation, are submitted before the application deadline.

As you prepare your application, remember that each program seeks candidates who are passionate, dedicated, and demonstrate a strong commitment to REI. Tailor your application to highlight your experiences, accomplishments, and research interests in this subspecialty. By submitting a complete and polished application, you maximize your chances of securing interviews and advancing in the selection process.

Fellowship Interviews

Securing an interview for a Reproductive Endocrinology fellowship is an exciting opportunity to showcase your skills, personality, and passion for the field. This section provides guidance on how to prepare for fellowship interviews and navigate the interview process effectively. The decision to offer applicants interviews appears to be influenced by objective standardized test scores, as well as a threshold of academic productivity. These items are less predictive of matching once the interview process begins, indicating that other factors, such as performance during the interview day, may be more heavily weighted [3].

Once you receive interview invitations, promptly respond to confirm your attendance and express your enthusiasm for the opportunity. Follow the provided instructions to schedule your interviews, keeping in mind any travel or accommodation arrangements that may be necessary. Since the COVID-19 pandemic, many fellowships have shifted how they conduct interviews. Fellowship interviews can take various formats, including in-person interviews, virtual interviews, or a combination of both. Dress professionally for both in-person and virtual interviews. In virtual interviews, choose an appropriate, well-lit location free from distractions. Maintain good eye contact, speak clearly and confidently, and actively listen to the interviewers' questions. Demonstrate professionalism, respect, and enthusiasm throughout the interview process.

Thorough preparation is key to a successful fellowship interview. Research each program extensively, reviewing their website, faculty profiles, ongoing research, and recent publications. Gain familiarity with the program's specific strengths, research areas, and clinical offerings. Prepare thoughtful questions to ask during the interview to demonstrate your interest and engagement.

During the interview, expect questions related to your background, experiences, clinical interests, research experience, and career goals as they were enumerated on your application and CV. Be prepared to discuss specific cases, research projects, or clinical scenarios related to REI. Consider how you can highlight your strengths, adaptability, problem-solving skills, and ability to work in a team. Emphasize your interest and experience in research during the interview. Discuss any previous research projects, contributions to publications or presentations, and your future research goals. Articulate how you envision incorporating research into your career as a Reproductive Endocrinologist.

After the interview, send a personalized thank you note or email to each interviewer within a few days of the interview. Express your appreciation for the opportunity to interview and reiterate your interest in the fellowship program. This gesture demonstrates your professionalism and serves as a reminder of your positive impression.

If you are fortunate to receive multiple interview invitations, keep track of your interview experiences and impressions of each program. Reflect on the pros and cons of each program, considering factors such as location, curriculum, research opportunities, and overall fit with your career goals. Once interviews are complete, carefully evaluate each program and make an informed decision when ranking your preferred programs.

Remember that fellowship interviews are a two-way process. While the program evaluates you as a candidate, it is also an opportunity for you to assess the program's compatibility with your goals and expectations. Remain confident, genuine, and enthusiastic throughout the interview process, and trust that your preparation and dedication will shine through.

The Fellowship Match Process

After completing the fellowship interviews, OB/GYN residents interested in REI must navigate the fellowship match process. The fellowship match process follows a structured algorithm through the National Resident Matching Program (NRMP). Applicants submit their rank order list of preferred programs, while programs submit their rank order list of preferred candidates. The algorithm then matches applicants with programs based on their preferences and available positions.

When creating your rank order list, carefully consider your preferences, including program reputation, location, curriculum, research opportunities, and personal factors. It is essential to prioritize programs where you feel you would thrive and receive comprehensive training. Seek advice from mentors, program directors, or current fellows to gather insights about specific programs.

Conclusion

Pursuing a fellowship in REI offers OB/GYN residents a unique opportunity to specialize in a field dedicated to reproductive health, fertility, and assisted reproductive technologies. Throughout this chapter, we have explored the fellowship application process, fellowship interviews, and the fellowship match process. By following the guidance provided and investing time and effort into each step, you can enhance your chances of securing a fellowship position in REI.

The journey towards a fellowship in REI requires dedication, perseverance, and a genuine passion for advancing reproductive healthcare. It is essential to research fellowship programs thoroughly, prepare a strong application, and approach interviews with confidence and professionalism. Remember to be authentic and let your enthusiasm for the field shine through.

References

1. Gambone JC, Segars JH, Cedars M, Schlaff WD. Fellowship training and board certification in reproductive endocrinology and infertility. Fertil Steril. 2015;104(1):3–7.
2. Society for Reproductive Endocrinology and Infertility (www.socrei.org).
3. Franasiak J, Kaser D, Goodman L, Patounakis G, Juneau C, Morin S, Neal S, Schlaff W, Scott R. Characterization of reproductive endocrinology and infertility (REI) fellowship applicants: guiding our mentees toward success. Fertil Res Pract. 2017;3:18.

Chapter 7
Urogynecology and Reconstructive Pelvic Surgery

Shayan Khorsandi

Introduction

Urogynecology, a subspecialty at the intersection of gynecology, urology, and colorectal surgery, is dedicated to the assessment and management of pelvic floor disorders (PFDs) that predominantly affect women. These disorders include urinary incontinence, fecal incontinence, pelvic organ prolapse, and a myriad of related conditions that can have a profound impact on a woman's quality of life [1]. The field of urogynecology has witnessed remarkable growth and recognition in recent years due to the increasing prevalence of PFDs and the demand for specialized care. As a result, urogynecology fellowships have emerged as critical to the training of healthcare professionals dedicated to improving the lives of women suffering from these conditions.

History

The roots of urogynecology can be traced back to the mid-twentieth century when physicians recognized the importance of addressing the complex interplay of pelvic floor structures. Early pioneers like Arnold Kegel and G. Plevnik laid the groundwork for understanding pelvic floor muscle function and dysfunction. However, it was not until the 1970s that healthcare professionals recognized the need for a specialized approach to pelvic floor disorders. The term "urogynecology" began to gain currency as the field expanded beyond traditional gynecology and urology, acknowledging the intricate interplay of pelvic structures. This paved the way to the creation of the American Urogynecologic Society (AUGS), founded in 1979. Since then, the

S. Khorsandi (✉)
Founder of Pelvic Solution Institute, Vega Baja, Puerto Rico

A. Malik et al. (eds.), *An Obstetrician/Gynecologist's Path*,
https://doi.org/10.1007/978-3-031-87098-9_7

society has played a crucial role in shaping urogynecology as a subspecialty [2]. AUGS, along with the International Urogynecological Association (IUGA), has been instrumental in establishing standards and guidelines for fellowship programs, promoting research, and advancing the education and training of urogynecologists.

As awareness of urogynecology has grown, so has the demand for specialized training. The 1980s and 1990s witnessed the establishment of urogynecology fellowships, providing a structured pathway for healthcare professionals to gain expertise in the assessment and management of pelvic floor disorders. In 2001, the American Board of Obstetrics and Gynecology (ABOG) introduced board certification in Female Pelvic Medicine and Reconstructive Surgery (FPMRS). This formal recognition further solidified urogynecology as a specialized field and emphasized the importance of standardized training [3].

Today, contemporary urogynecology is characterized by ongoing advancements in research and a strong emphasis on multidisciplinary collaboration. Urogynecologists collaborate with experts in urology, colorectal surgery, general gynecology, and other relevant fields to ensure comprehensive care for patients with pelvic floor disorders.

The Evolution of the Urogynecology Subspecialty's Name: Navigating Terminology Confusion

The nomenclature of the urogynecology subspecialty has undergone a fascinating evolution, reflecting a nuanced journey of defining its scope and expertise. Understanding the historical timeline may help provide clarity for all healthcare professionals, especially those still in residency thinking of applying for fellowship. In 1995, the subspecialty was introduced as "Urogynecology and Reconstructive Pelvic Surgery" (URPS), emphasizing both the urinary and gynecologic aspects of pelvic floor disorders with a focus on reconstructive interventions. The year 2000 marked a pivotal transition as the subspecialty shifted its name to "Female Pelvic Medicine and Reconstructive Surgery" (FPMRS), aiming for greater precision in reflecting the comprehensive nature of care, including broader aspects of pelvic medicine. In 2023, there was a notable shift back to the original name, "Urogynecology and Reconstructive Pelvic Surgery" (URPS), recognizing the historical significance of the term and aligning more closely with the evolving understanding of the field's breadth and depth.

The shifting nomenclature has at times created confusion, particularly among residents and healthcare professionals unfamiliar with the historical timeline. Initially, "urogynecology" was widely used, but with the transition to FPMRS in 2000, uncertainty emerged regarding the preferred term for the fellowship. This period witnessed a divergence in terminology. Embracing this evolution ensures that healthcare professionals can confidently navigate the terminological landscape, understanding that both "urogynecology," "URPS," and "FPMRS" are valid and historically rooted terms for this specialized field.

Application Process

Applying for urogynecology fellowships is a competitive process. Prospective candidates submit applications through centralized platforms like the Electronic Residency Application Service (ERAS) to the participating ACGME accredited urogynecology fellowship programs. These applications typically include a candidate's curriculum vitae, personal statement, three letters of recommendation (one normally from the residency program director), and 2nd and 3rd year CREOG scores.

For aspiring urogynecology fellows, the application timeline for the ERAS (Electronic Residency Application Service) is a crucial aspect to keep in mind. ERAS opens for application submission normally around mid-November, and the accurate timeline can be found at the American Urogynecological Society (AUGS) [4]. A mid-January date typically serves as the application deadline for consideration in the first round of interview offers by these programs.

If applicants submit their Urogynecology Fellowship application by the specified deadline, they will be eligible for consideration in the first round of interview offers.

The interview season for urogynecology programs kicks off officially in March, presenting applicants with the opportunity to showcase their credentials. It is crucial to meticulously adhere to key dates for a smooth application process and to maximize the chances of securing coveted interview opportunities in the competitive field of urogynecology fellowships. Additionally, carefully review the program descriptions you are applying to. While most programs admit one fellow per year, some have a mix of urology and obgyn. These programs may alternate their selection process each year, accepting a urologist one year and an obgyn the next. The comprehensive list of all ACGME accredited programs, along with their respective program directors, is available on the AUGS website [5] (https://www.augs.org/assets/1/1/PublicListProgramsBySpecialty_22-23.pdf).

Fellowship Training

Urogynecology fellowship programs typically last two years for those with a urology residency background and three years for those with an obgyn residency background. The first year is dedicated to intensive clinical training, exposing fellows to diverse cases of pelvic floor disorders [1]. Fellows develop expertise in evaluating, diagnosing, and managing these conditions across outpatient and inpatient settings.

Surgical proficiency is a fundamental aspect of urogynecology fellowship training. Fellows actively participate in and, under supervision, perform various urogynecological procedures, including pelvic reconstructive surgery, minimally invasive surgeries, and urodynamic evaluations. Surgical skills are crucial as many patients with pelvic floor disorders may require surgical interventions [3].

In addition to clinical and surgical training, urogynecology fellows engage in didactic education. This comprehensive component includes regular lectures, seminars, journal clubs, and multidisciplinary conferences covering pelvic floor anatomy, physiology, pathophysiology, medical management, and the latest research in the field [6].

The structure of the subspecialty-specific fellowship program in Urogynecology and Reconstructive Pelvic Surgery spans 24 months. The program focuses on providing 18 months of hands-on clinical activity, allowing fellows to gain proficiency in managing female pelvic disorders. Protected research time, a vital component lasting 12 months, allows fellows to concentrate on research projects during the week, with each program adopting different strategies for managing this dedicated time.

For OBGYN graduates, the program emphasizes research methodologies and scholarly contributions. An appointed faculty research mentor guides fellows through the research curriculum, covering research design, methodology, data analysis, and grant writing. Each fellow is required to complete and defend a scholarly paper (thesis) meeting certification standards.

Urology graduates follow a similar educational track, developing a scholarly manuscript or quality improvement project paper. This project demonstrates proficiency in research design, methodology, and analysis. Before completing the fellowship, each urology graduate presents their scholarly project orally, with the goal of contributing meaningfully to the scientific discourse in female pelvic medicine and reconstructive surgery [1].

Fellows gain exposure to both inpatient and outpatient settings, taking supervised responsibility for comprehensive patient care, including evaluation, diagnosis, therapy selection, and complication management. Continuity of patient care, spanning preoperative to post-operative settings and inpatient contacts, ensures a holistic understanding of patient management. The didactic component of the URPS fellowship programs complements clinical and research aspects.

During the fellowship program, some institutions allow fellows to engage in independent practice within their core specialty. However, this participation should not exceed 20% of their weekly schedule or extend beyond 10 weeks in an academic year, aligning with ACGME regulations (equivalent to 4 h per week). Other programs offer opportunities for global health work or involvement and the flexibility to pursue additional scholarly activities, such as obtaining a master's degree.

What to Look for in a Program

Selecting the right urogynecology fellowship program is a significant decision that requires careful consideration. Your choice should align with your career goals and preferred learning style.

Prioritize programs offering immersive clinical training, especially in the first year of fellowship. Exposure to diverse cases in varied settings, including both outpatient and inpatient scenarios, is essential for developing proficiency in evaluating, diagnosing, and managing pelvic floor disorders [1].

Surgical proficiency is a fundamental aspect of urogynecology fellowship training. Look for a program that provides a diverse set of tools for effectively managing complex pelvic cases. A comprehensive understanding of various treatment modalities enhances your preparedness for real-world scenarios. Evaluate whether the program facilitates active participation and decision-making during urogynecological procedures. Programs that offer opportunities to guide residents and medical students of diverse backgrounds significantly contribute to your development as a surgeon. Fellowship programs that incorporate a blend of surgical backgrounds also provide a unique perspective on surgery. Positive characteristics include collaborative efforts between urology, urogynecology, colorectal, dermatology, pelvic floor physical therapists, and sexual health educators. Such collaborations contribute to shaping your skills as both a surgeon and clinician.

Consider the didactic component of the program, which includes lectures, seminars, and conferences. An ideal program covers a comprehensive range of topics relevant to female pelvic medicine and reconstructive surgery, enriching your educational experience [6].

Examine the program's structure, ensuring a substantial period (at least 18 months) is dedicated to hands-on clinical experience. Protected research time, spanning 12 months, is key for those keen on contributing to the advancement of the field. Be aware that the management of this research time may vary among programs.

For OBGYN graduates, assess the program's commitment to supporting educational endeavors in research, global health opportunities or pursuing a master's degree. Evaluate your research skills and the level of mentoring required to develop your thesis. Investigate whether the program provides additional research resources (such as a statistician) to enhance your understanding of conducting an appropriate thesis. Completing and defending a scholarly paper is a significant component of this fellowship [3].

Lastly, gauge the program's overall environment by seeking insights from current or past fellows. Their experiences offer valuable perspectives on the work environment, mentorship, and overall satisfaction. It is crucial to remember that fellowship programs foster a closer teaching experience than in the past, allowing you to develop personal relationships with attendings and professionals who may become an extended family. Choose a program aligned with your views and values.

By meticulously weighing these factors, you can tailor your choice to align with your career goals, learning preferences, and the unique offerings of each urogynecology fellowship program. Urogynecology, by its nature, is multidisciplinary. Programs that encourage collaboration with other specialties will better prepare you for comprehensive patient care [1].

Certification and Accreditation

Upon successful completion of the urogynecology fellowship, graduates can pursue board certification through the American Board of Obstetrics and Gynecology (ABOG). For gynecologists, this process involves a familiarized two-step approach. Initially, qualification for the written exam, known as the Qualifying exam, is attained upon fellowship program completion. Subsequently, eligibility for the Certifying exam is granted. This comprises an oral examination, during which candidates must upload their case list and fellowship thesis. Additionally, candidates are required to defend their thesis during this process.

Lifestyle

Embarking on a career in urogynecology offers a profound opportunity to influence women's health and enhance their quality of life. Beyond the inherent satisfaction of making a meaningful impact, urogynecology provides an extraordinary level of flexibility, allowing practitioners to tailor their career to align with personal aspirations and lifestyle preferences. Whether one's passion lies in research, entrepreneurial ventures through private practice, academic pursuits, or industry engagement, urogynecology accommodates diverse interests. The field's dynamism and constant innovation cater to those seeking a continuously evolving and growing professional landscape, addressing the expanding healthcare needs of a larger population. The journey in urogynecology not only promises a fulfilling professional life but also empowers individuals to craft a career that resonates with their unique lifestyle and ambitions.

References

1. Gerjevic KA, Brandes E, Gormley EA, Auty SG, Strohbehn K. Trends among female pelvic medicine and reconstructive surgery fellowships and graduates. Female Pelvic Med Reconstr Surg. 2022;28(6):e211–4. https://doi.org/10.1097/SPV.0000000000001186.
2. American Urogynecology Society. History. Available at: https://www.augs.org/about/history/ Accessed on 30 Dec 2023.
3. Steers WD. Establishing the subspecialty of female pelvic medicine and reconstructive surgery in the United States of America. Arab J Urol. 2013;11(2):113–6. https://doi.org/10.1016/j.aju.2013.01.003.
4. American Urogynecology Society. Key Dates. Available at: https://www.augs.org/education/fellowship-application-key-dates. Accessed on 30 Dec 2023.
5. American Urogynecology Society. Programs Lis. Available at: https://www.augs.org/assets/1/1/PublicListProgramsBySpecialty_22-23.pdf. Accessed on 30 Dec 2023.
6. Mishra K, Lopes VV, Hampton BS. Global health interest among female pelvic medicine and reconstructive surgery fellows. J Reprod Med. 2015;60(11-12):501–6.

Chapter 8
Complex Family Planning

Carolyn Ross

Introduction

The Fellowship in Complex Family Planning (CFP) was started in 1991 in an effort to combat the "graying of abortion providers." The goal was to train a new generation of obstetrician-gynecologists who could provide complex abortion and contraception care to patients, and become experts in the field of Family Planning. The fellowship became accredited by the Accreditation Council for Graduate Medical Education (ACGME) in 2019. There are currently 35 fellowship programs available for applicants to choose from, with the number of fellowships growing every year as more programs seek and receive accreditation. The fellowship in CFP is a two-year commitment, with one year focusing on clinical training and the second year focusing on research endeavors and elective time. There are many important considerations when applying to CFP fellowship, which will be detailed in this chapter.

Application

Applicants may apply for CFP fellowship through the Electronic Residency Application Service (ERAS) and will participate in the match through the National Residency Matching Program (NRMP). Most applicants will apply during their third year of residency if they wish to matriculate immediately after finishing residency. However, some applicants may choose to work as generalists before deciding that they would like to pursue fellowship in CFP. Applications open in the fall and

C. Ross (✉)
Department of Obstetrics and Gynecology, Cooper Medical School of Rowan University and Cooper University Health Care, Camden, NJ, USA

A. Malik et al. (eds.), *An Obstetrician/Gynecologist's Path*,
https://doi.org/10.1007/978-3-031-87098-9_8

interviews take place between June and August. Match day occurs in September with matriculation the following summer.

Choosing a Fellowship

The CFP Fellowship focuses on providing training for fellows in complex abortion care, so all fellows will obtain the necessary experience to become abortion providers through at least the second trimester of pregnancy. Due to differing state restrictions on abortion, some fellowship sites may require fellows to travel out of state for necessary training in later abortion care. Applicants should inquire about the scope of abortion training available at each site—whether all of the abortions are done in-hospital or whether they will also train at an outside clinic, either in-state or out-of-state. The applicant should gain an understanding of how state policy changes have impacted clinical training and what each fellowship site is doing to ensure that fellows receive adequate surgical volume. Certain fellowship sites may also provide opportunities to learn feticidal injection or moderate sedation for procedures. Fellows will also gain comfort with complex contraception, both with choosing birth control for the medically complex patient and dealing with technically challenging implant and IUD insertions and removals.

Research is an exciting and integral component of CFP Fellowship. Each fellow is expected to complete a research project by the end of fellowship and present it at the annual research meeting. When choosing a fellowship, one should consider the research strengths of each site. Some may have more developed research infrastructures than others, and some may have access to different patient populations of interest (i.e., patients with substance use disorders, incarcerated patients, adolescent patients, etc.). Applicants should consider if they are interested in qualitative, quantitative, or mixed methods research and should have an idea of a project that they might be interested in working on when applying for fellowship. Sites may vary in that they might have an established project that they will want the fellow to pursue versus having the option to begin a new project.

The CFP Fellowship is unique in that there are oftentimes generalist duties for fellows in addition to the research project and providing abortion/contraceptive care for patients. The applicant should inquire about what type of generalist work he or she will be expected to perform while in fellowship. If an applicant is interested in continuing to perform major surgeries or do obstetrics, he or she should find out the opportunities that are available at each fellowship site. Moonlighting is sometimes possible and taking call is often a requirement, although what call looks like at different institutions may vary widely (e.g., holding the Family Planning pager, covering L&D, gyn-of-the-week, etc.).

Fellowship Experience

The CFP Fellowship is a two-year program. One year will focus on clinical training—abortion and miscarriage care for complex and second trimester patients as well as complex contraception training. The second year focuses on research, with time for electives. Program sites may vary in structure.

During fellowship, fellows will complete a Master of Science or Public Health or other equivalent degree to gain education in study design, statistics and epidemiology, manuscript and grant writing, and research ethics. This will inform the research project that the fellow completes and will prepare them to become leaders in the field.

Fellows should consider their ultimate career goals during their training. Graduated fellows will be well equipped to start a new Ryan program at an institution needing training for residents, start a Fellowship, work as a medical director for Planned Parenthood or another independent clinic, travel to provide abortion care in underserved areas, and much more. Fellows may participate in advocacy training through Physicians for Reproductive Health's Leadership Training Academy and are required to complete a minimum two-week block rotation in a low-resource family planning setting during their two years of fellowship. There are many opportunities for CFP Fellows that will prepare them for the workforce.

Board Certification

Since becoming certified by the ACGME and ABOG, CFP Fellowship requires a qualifying (CFP "written boards") exam followed by a certifying (CFP "oral boards") exam. The qualifying exam is a multiple-choice test covering the following topics:

Contraception (35%)
Early Pregnancy Evaluation and Management (15%)
Abortion/Pregnancy Termination (40%)
Research, Health Policy, and Advocacy (5%)
Core Competencies and Cross Content (5%)

The qualifying exam is administered at the end of July, and the certifying exam is administered in Dallas, Texas, in April.

Conclusions

Complex Family Planning is an exciting field in which to pursue fellowship training. As the national landscape continues to change, more obstetrician-gynecologists will answer the call to provide safe and effective family planning for their patients and will pursue fellowship. As CFP is now ACGME-certified, it will continue to grow as a competitive subspecialty.

References

1. www.abog.org
2. www.acgme.org

Chapter 9
Minimally Invasive Gynecologic Surgery Fellowship

Lauren Spivack

History of the Fellowship

Starting in the 1980s and 1990s, as laparoscopic gynecologic surgery took off, one-year reproductive surgery fellowships were first established without any specific affiliation to existing organizations. These were born out of the concern that most OB/GYN residents were not fully trained in modern laparoscopic procedures, even by the time of graduation [1]. In 2001, the American Association of Gynecologic Laparoscopists (AAGL) and Society for Reproductive Science (SRS) joined together to officially establish the Fellowship in Minimally Invasive Gynecologic Surgery (FMIGS). It included a specified curriculum as well as required research. Eventually, the FMIGS fellowship became affiliated solely with AAGL. To date, there are 600+ fellows that have completed the AAGL FMIGS Fellowship. Per the AAGL website, "the overall goal of the fellowship is for graduates to serve as an independent specialist and consultant in the medical and surgical management and techniques of advanced, benign, complex gynecologic conditions at a level surpassing competence expected by completion of a categorical residency" [2].

Application Process

Those who are eligible for an FMIGS Fellowship must have completed an ACGME-accredited OB/GYN residency. The goal of the fellowship is to enhance gynecologic training through advancing knowledge and surgical skills for complex benign gynecologic cases. This is because many residents complete OB/GYN residency

L. Spivack (✉)
Department of Obstetrics and Gynecology, Rowan-Virtua School of Osteopathic Medicine, Stratford, NJ, USA

A. Malik et al. (eds.), *An Obstetrician/Gynecologist's Path*,
https://doi.org/10.1007/978-3-031-87098-9_9

without sufficient laparoscopic skills for more complex cases. Although the training is standardized by way of required research and minimum surgical cases by type, each program is slightly different, with varying degrees of focus on robotic surgery versus laparoscopic surgery, urogynecologic procedures, exposure to gynecologic oncology, as well as specialization in pelvic pain. There is a comprehensive website (https://aagl.org/fmigs-programs/) which gives extensive information on the fellowship and each individual program.

There are currently 60 fellowship programs. There are 54 fellowship sites in the USA, 3 in Canada, 1 in Brazil, 1 in Colombia, 1 in Mexico, and 1 in Ireland. Although there are 60 programs, there are several programs (18 in 2024) that are not participating in the match in any given year. This number changes slightly year to year based on the availability of fellowship positions.

Programs typically accept anywhere from one to three fellows, some on an annual basis and some every other year, depending on case volume at the site. Application to the fellowship occurs during PGY-3 and 4 year.

Specific due dates for applications and interview schedules will vary year to year. However, the application deadline is usually around the 1st of May. The non-refundable application fee ($350.00 in 2024) is due at the same time. At the end of May, the first wave of interview invites are sent to applicants. The deadline for candidates to accept or decline the interview invitations is typically one week after that, at which point there is a second wave of interview notifications. Interviews usually take place from June to September. There is an interview schedule calendar on the AAGL website listing each program's interview dates—typically programs have a few days of interviews. After submitting a match list, the applicant will be notified in late September if they have matched to a program.

Application Requirements

Requirements for application to the fellowship that are posted on the AAGL website include:

1. Digital, high-resolution, headshot photo (300 dpi). Headshot photos will be forwarded to the programs, after an interview has been offered. These photos will be used for AAGL/FMIGS media platforms.
2. Curriculum Vitae. This includes your educational pedigree, all abstracts, and presentations at regional and national meetings, publications, honors, awards, and achievements.
3. Three letters of reference. One letter should be from your residency director. The letters of reference must be submitted directly to the Fellowship office by e-mail: fmigs@aagl.org. Letters should be addressed to *Program Director* or *To Whom It May Concern*. Additional letters may be submitted. Letters must be submitted by no later than May 1.
4. Your residency ACGME case list brief summary (1 page).

5. Personal statement discussing your interest in pursuing MIGS training (1 page max, size 10 font/single space).
6. CREOG Scores. Include all available scores and not only the highest.
7. ECFMG certificate (if applicable).
8. TOEFL IBT certificate (if applicable).
9. Official copy of USMLE or LCCE transcript. Submit to the Fellowship office by e-mail fmigs@aagl.org or surface mail at 6757 Katella Avenue, Cypress, CA 90630.
10. If you are currently not a resident in training, please provide the following:
    - A description of your current practice.
    - A list of all hospital staff and teaching appointments currently held, including types of privileges.
    - A copy of your malpractice policy[1].

At the conclusion of the interview process, the rank list is due (again, the date may vary year to year). The results of the match are posted in September, and the applicant will find out if they have been selected into a program.

Similar to medical school and residency applications, there is much information and documentation to be gathered. It is important to give ample time to do this, especially requesting letters of recommendation.

Components of Training

FMIGS training includes clinical training (surgical planning and pre- and post-operative care), significant surgical experience (varies based on program regarding the balance of laparoscopic versus robotic versus vaginal hysteroscopic surgery), didactics, resident and medical student teaching responsibilities, research requirements, and variable on call responsibilities.

There is a surgical competency list which includes minimum case numbers that must be completed in order to complete the training. Per the AAGL website, "the FMIGS Surgical Competency List must be used and completed for each fellow by the end of the fellowship training. Surgical procedures available for the fellow must include but are not limited to: diagnostic and operative hysteroscopy, diagnostic and operative laparoscopy, laparotomy, robotic surgery, and ambulatory procedures. Additionally, the program must ensure fellow competency by experience and/or simulation in multiple types of vaginal surgery (e.g., prolapse repair, vaginal tissue extraction, vaginal septums, vNOTES) including vaginal hysterectomy, the management of small and large bowel concerns as it relates to complex gynecologic disease, and gynecologic conditions that may impact fertility (e.g., uterine septum, intrauterine adhesions, and uterine leiomyomas)." [3]

There are minimum case numbers to be reached, allowing for the breadth and depth of benign gynecologic surgeries, focusing on minimally invasive surgical modalities. Additionally, some programs may have a particular focus on areas like pelvic pain.

On the AAGL website, there is detailed information for each program as to length of the fellowship (2 years versus 3 years), whether the program is accepting applications in that application cycle, information on faculty, case volume and type, didactic schedule, OB and GYN coverage responsibilities, and research.

The research requirement includes completion of one course in clinical research, research design, biostatistics, or epidemiology unless the fellow has coursework within the last 10 years that is graduate level. This requirement can be completed in a classroom or online setting. The research project must be an independent research project with the requirement of a mentor and IRB approval if necessitated by the type of study. It must be original research and can be a systematic review or a meta-analysis, but must ultimately be submitted for publication in a peer-reviewed journal prior to completion of the fellowship.

What to Look for in a Program

The AAGL website lists all of the programs with program specific summaries that the applicant will find pertinent to deciding what program fits their individual goals.

The applicant must decide if they want a program that is focused exclusively on laparoscopy or one that is more balanced between robotics and laparoscopy. Additionally, the applicant should assess whether vaginal surgery is an important surgical skill set they wish to have, and whether they value more of a urogynecologic focus or even more of a gynecologic oncology focus. If the applicant desires more hysteroscopy experience, there are programs with faculty that focus on this as well. Each program has a detailed case log of prior fellows' completed surgeries. This is important for an applicant to review during the interview process to decide if they would like to train there or not. Many of these details can be found in the descriptions of the program and can also be inquired about during the interview process. It should be noted how many fellows there are in the program (range of 1–4) and how frequently fellows are accepted (yearly or every other year), as one option may be more preferable to a given applicant. It should also be noted whether there has been any recent difficulty with obtaining the minimum case requirements for graduation and how this is handled if the problem should arise.

Additionally, there are programs in which the fellow will function as more of a junior attending in the second years of fellowship, or will take obstetric call (in or out of house), gynecologic call, and/or MIGS call. Factoring in future career goals can be helpful in determining what the applicant might want their fellowship to look like.

What You Can Do After MIGS Fellowship

After completion of a minimally invasive gynecologic surgery fellowship, one will have the option of practicing as a General OB/GYN, a MIGS surgeon, or some combination of both. If the goal is to be exclusively a MIGS surgeon, it is absolutely possible after completion of the fellowship. It can at times be difficult to find positions where no obstetrics is required, but they do exist and are likely to become more prevalent. There also exists the possibility of starting out doing some office obstetrics and/or obstetrical call, and then transitioning to GYN/MIGS only as surgical volume increases. If the intention is to practice only GYN/MIGS, referrals from general OB/GYNs in the area will be important. Networking early in one's career and volunteering to take on difficult cases from fellow colleagues can help in establishing a steady referral network.

References

1. AAGL website: https://survey.alchemer.com/s3/7616964/Fellow-Application-2025-Appointments
2. Thomas R, Haynes S. Minimally invasive surgery fellowship. In: Yoon-Flannery K, Fisher C, Neff M, editors. A surgeon's path. Cham: Springer; 2018. https://doi.org/10.1007/978-3-319-78846-3_9.
3. https://survey.alchemer.com/s3/7616964/Fellow-Application-2025-Appointments AAGL website.

Chapter 10
Pediatric and Adolescent Gynecology

Beth I. Schwartz

Introduction

Pediatric and adolescent gynecology (PAG) is a newer subspecialty of Obstetrics and Gynecology that focuses on gynecologic problems in individuals from birth into young adulthood. This field was created with the acknowledgement both that children and adolescents often have to be approached and treated differently than adults and that this population has a unique set of medical and surgical issues that are often unfamiliar to most obstetricians and gynecologists. These concerns include complex hormonal problems, prepubertal vulvovaginal concerns, and congenital genitourinary anomalies. PAGs also frequently work in multidisciplinary teams to care for patients with bleeding disorders, those undergoing treatment for or survivors of cancer, gender diverse youth, and patients with anorectal malformations and disorders of sex development. Fellowship training focuses on exposure to this patient population and both common and rare medical and surgical diagnoses, as well as collaborative multidisciplinary evaluation and treatment for complex patients and medical conditions. Because PAG is such a small field, there is a wonderful sense of community with frequent clinical and research collaboration and opportunities for advocacy. While PAG is not currently an official ACGME-accredited fellowship program within Obstetrics and Gynecology, there is now an ABOG PAG Focused Practice Designation to provide recognition and improve ongoing professional development for this subspecialty.

B. I. Schwartz (✉)
Department of Obstetrics and Gynecology, Thomas Jefferson University, Philadelphia, PA, USA

Division of Adolescent Medicine and Pediatric Gynecology, Nemours Children's Health, Wilmington, DE, USA

A. Malik et al. (eds.), *An Obstetrician/Gynecologist's Path*,
https://doi.org/10.1007/978-3-031-87098-9_10

The Path to Fellowship

As most Obstetrics and Gynecology departments and residency programs do not have a pediatric and adolescent gynecologist, the majority of medical students and Ob/Gyn residents do not have significant exposure to this field during their training. However, they may realize that they get excited when a teenager comes to the office to discuss birth control or remember the child with persistent vaginal itching on their Pediatrics rotation or the adolescent with primary amenorrhea on their Reproductive Endocrinology and Infertility elective. If you recognize that you like working with this patient population or are fascinated by their medical conditions, it is important to try to get more exposure to the field during medical school or residency. If there is a PAG provider in your department or hospital, spend as much time with that person as possible, either within your existing rotations or through an elective. If your department or hospital does not have a PAG provider, reach out to someone in your city or region or even nationally by email. We are a very friendly group who often know firsthand how difficult it is to forge a path that no one around you has done before. Many of us have mentored students and residents locally and nationally who do not have access to a local PAG provider. For those with minimal or no PAG exposure during residency, it would be beneficial to do an away elective at a program with a PAG fellowship. This will allow three things to occur: (1) exposure to the breadth of work and lifestyle of PAG to make sure that you are interested in this subspecialty, (2) introduction to and hopeful involvement in a PAG-related research project, and (3) networking and ability to obtain a letter of recommendation from a well-known person in the field, ideally a fellowship program director.

Fellowship programs recognize that not all applicants have adequate exposure to PAG during residency and that not all applicants are able to do away rotations. The most important thing is to demonstrate your interest and that you have exposed yourself to the field as much as possible. This could include talking to current PAG fellows and attendings, attending regional or national meetings, and getting involved with PAG research. If you cannot do a true PAG research project at your institution, think about doing one with an adjacent population (e.g., pregnant teens, young adults with primary ovarian insufficiency, adults with disabilities); writing a review article or a systematic review on a PAG topic; or being involved with PAG research remotely, such as secondary analysis of an existing data set.

Do I Need to Do a Fellowship?

This is a frequent question about Pediatric and Adolescent Gynecology: "Do I really need to do an entire fellowship just to prescribe birth control to a 15-year-old?" Absolutely not. But that is really not what PAG is about. If your goals are to see a patient population that others often would prefer to avoid, you likely do not have to do a fellowship. You can join a practice and make it known that you want to see all the teens. However, while adolescent contraception and menstrual management may be the "bread and butter" of PAG, there is much more to the field. Without any specialty training, would you feel comfortable counseling about and managing hormonal contraception for a 12-year-old nonverbal, nonambulatory patient with a syndrome you have never heard of who sees 5 specialists at the regional children's hospital and has a page-long medication list? What about a 3-year-old with persistent vaginal itching that her pediatrician has struggled to manage? Or a 13-year-old with primary amenorrhea and absent pubertal development due to Turner syndrome or after a bone marrow transplant for her ALL? Would you feel comfortable operating on a patient with hematocolpos due to a transverse vaginal septum or a newborn in the NICU with a cloaca? These are the conditions that the fellowship is intended to treat, as well as to support research about these rare conditions and provide advocacy for adolescents and traditionally underserved populations. So if you just want to see uncomplicated teens, then you likely do not have to do a fellowship, but if you want to be part of multidisciplinary teams caring for complex patients in a children's hospital, then you do.

How to Choose a Fellowship Program

Once you have decided that you want to do a PAG fellowship, how do you choose a program? The geographical location and length of the program may be important factors. While most programs are 2 years, a few are only 1. Others provide the choice of 1 vs. 2 years, with the opportunity to obtain a Master's degree during the extra year in fields such as Public Health, Higher Education, Clinical Translational Research, or Health Informatics. Your choice of program will likely also be influenced by your clinical and research interests and planned practice composition and setting after fellowship. Some applicants may want to practice PAG as part of a general Ob/Gyn practice and thus may benefit most from a program with good exposure to "bread and butter" PAG. Others may plan to pursue a career in complex vaginal reconstruction and will thus value a high-volume surgical program with specialty multidisciplinary teams for complex, rare congenital anomalies.

The amount and type of research training, protected research time, research infrastructure and support, and current research areas of interest may be important to some applicants but not to others. You may identify certain attendings as important clinical and research mentors. Lastly, the call schedule and division of labor between fellows with residents and attendings is also something to consider, both in terms of clinical experience and lifestyle. An away elective rotation can be extremely useful in helping identify clinical interests, program culture and lifestyle, and what aspects of fellowship are most important to you.

Application and Interview Process

Pediatric and Adolescent Gynecology is a small subspecialty, but the fellowships have grown in both number and size over time. There are currently 16 fellowship programs in North America: 13 in the United States and 3 in Canada. Most programs have 1 open spot each year, but some only take 1 fellow every other year and a few programs take 2 fellows per year. As such, the number of available spots changes each year.

All programs accept a simple common application. In addition to this application, other requirements are a current curriculum vitae; at least 3 letters of recommendation, one of which must be from the Director of your residency training program; a copy of your medical school diploma; ECFMG and TOEFL IBT certificates, if applicable; an official copy of your USMLE or LCCE transcript; and a personal statement of career goals, with discussion of how you plan to use this fellowship training. Some programs may have additional requirements. Information about each of the fellowship programs, requirements, and contacts can be found on the North American Society for Pediatric and Adolescent Gynecology (NASPAG) website under the Education tab and Fellowships.

Applications are accepted each year between March 31 and July 5, with interviews over the summer. PAG fellowship programs participate in the NRMP matching service according to the Ob/Gyn Fellowship Match Schedule, which occurs in October. All fellowship programs start in July.

Fellowship Training

The structure and the content of each fellowship program is different, but all include a combination of outpatient clinics, inpatient consults or service, surgery, education, and research. There is typically participation in multidisciplinary programs, such as with Hematology for menstrual management of patients with suspected or diagnosed bleeding disorders; Oncology for oncofertility and reproductive survivorship; Dermatology for vulvar dermatoses; various specialties for care of transgender and gender diverse youth; Urology and Surgery for anorectal malformations; and Endocrinology, Urology, and Genetics for disorders of sex development. Fellows may also spend time rotating with other specialties.

Education on PAG topics is often done through a fellows' lecture series within their division and from other subspecialties. There are also regular lectures in conjunction with other PAG fellows nationally on clinical and research topics by leaders in the field. Twice a year, there is a NASPAG Fellows' Boot Camp with a half- or full-day of lectures for all current PAG fellows, as well as fellows in Adolescent Medicine and possibly other subspecialties.

All fellows must complete a research project. This can take a variety of forms. Fellows often join existing projects or start their own, based on their clinical interests. PAG fellows are also active participants in multisite research projects through the NASPAG Research Network. Fellows regularly have oral and poster presentations at the NASPAG Annual Clinical and Research Meeting.

Lifestyle during fellowship is based on a variety of factors, including the clinical and surgical volume, call schedule, and culture of the program. Call at all programs is home telephone call, but who takes first call and how often fellows are called and have to come in overnight and on weekends vary between programs. The most common surgical emergencies are adnexal torsion, straddle injuries, and labial abscesses. Overall, regardless of the exact program and schedule, life during PAG fellowship is generally much kinder and gentler than during Ob/Gyn residency.

Attending Life

Life as a PAG attending depends significantly on the job, practice setting, and the individual's career goals and ambitions. Most PAGs work in academic medical centers and teach medical students and residents as part of their jobs, but there are a few who work in solo or multispecialty private practice. Some physicians practice PAG as a niche area within the scope of a general Ob/Gyn practice, but most do not. Very few recent fellowship graduates continue to practice Obstetrics, although some run Teen Ob clinics or take some Labor and Delivery call. While most current PAG providers see only pediatric patients, some continue to practice adult Gynecology in general or may see a subset of adult patients with complex medical or surgical conditions. Some of these factors depend on whether the position is at a children's hospital, an adult hospital, or a combination.

Call schedule is often a major contributor to lifestyle. PAG call is almost exclusively home call, but the frequency of call and what it entails vary. Does the job include answering patient and parent calls? Do you have to go into the hospital for admissions, consults, and surgeries? Will you be the only one who takes PAG call or will you split it with partners, Pediatric Surgery, adult Gynecology, or Adolescent Medicine? Do you take adult Gynecology or Labor and Delivery call? On a related note, how does call affect your salary or reimbursement structure?

While there is a wide range in the scope of practice and day-to-day schedule of a pediatric and adolescent gynecologist, this field offers an opportunity to care for underserved populations with unique medical, surgical, and psychosocial challenges. There is ample opportunity for research on both common and rare conditions in a nascent field. It also offers entrance into a tight-knit community with unparalleled collegiality and a good sense of humor and fun.

References

1. North American Society for Pediatric and Adolescent Gynecology Fellowships: https://naspag.memberclicks.net/PAGFellowship
2. American Board of Obstetrics and Gynecology Pediatric and Adolescent Gynecology Focused Practice Designation: https://www.abog.org/maintenance-of-certification/focused-practice-designation/pediatric-and-adolescent-gynecology/overview

Chapter 11
Nontraditional Fellowships in Obstetrics and Gynecology (Ob/Gyn)

Laura Zalles and Latisha Moreta

What Are Nontraditional Fellowships?

Nontraditional fellowships encompass formal training for graduated Ob/Gyn residents in a field that is not certified by the American Board of Obstetrics and Gynecology (ABOG). Some of these specialties, such as Critical Care or Medical Genetics, have fellowships that are accredited by the Accreditation Council for Graduate Medical Education (ACGME) and/or allow for additional board certification. Others, such as Global Health or Hospitalist/Laborist fellowships, solely provide focused training for career development within Ob/Gyn. In this chapter, we will review some nontraditional fellowships, advantages of pursuing them, and what a career after a nontraditional fellowship might look like.

Who Pursues Nontraditional Fellowships?

There are many different reasons to pursue a nontraditional fellowship. Residency is standardized to train well-rounded general Obstetricians and Gynecologists. Outside of core Ob/Gyn competencies, exposure to the many facades of women's health is dependent on the training setting. The location, size, patient population, and faculty interests of a training program will influence resident experiences. Many general Ob/Gyns use nontraditional fellowships to allow for structured mentorship in a focused area of Ob/Gyn that he/she/they had limited exposure to in residency.

L. Zalles (✉)
Division of Reproductive Endocrinology and Infertility, University of Colorado, Boulder, CO, USA

L. Moreta
NYC Health and Hospitals, Jacobi Medical Center, Bronx, NY, USA

A. Malik et al. (eds.), *An Obstetrician/Gynecologist's Path*,
https://doi.org/10.1007/978-3-031-87098-9_11

This additional time provides high-volume training in a more specialized focus as well as mentorship by people who have also focused their careers on a subspecialty. Upon graduation, fellows may be more marketable and well connected in the focus of their choice, as these very specialized fields tend to be smaller professional networks.

Additionally, a nontraditional fellowship can often completely alter the practice of graduated fellows, allowing for interdisciplinary specialization. For example, there are Ob/Gyn Clinical Geneticists who apply their combined skill sets in areas such as preconception or perinatal genetic testing, disorders of sex development, and the management of inborn errors of metabolism in pregnancy. Similarly, a fellowship in Breast Surgery would allow an Ob/Gyn graduate to develop a practice spanning gynecologic and breast care, or to pivot away from traditional Ob/Gyn and focus solely on breast surgery.

Other times, residents choose to pursue a nontraditional fellowship while preparing to apply for a competitive traditional ABOG fellowship—for example, a Critical Care fellowship in preparation for Maternal Fetal Medicine (MFM) or a Medical Genetics fellowship in preparation for Reproductive Endocrinology and Infertility. Many MFM fellowship programs even provide the opportunity for dual training in Medical Genetics with an additional year; however, this track is typically pursued while applying directly to MFM fellowship. Other examples of nontraditional fellowships include:

Critical Care
Global Health/Global Surgery
Hospitalist/Laborist
Medical Justice and Advocacy
Reproductive Medicine and Immunology
Quality and Safety in Women's Health
Women's Health Equity
Breast Surgery
Sexual Medicine
Academic Specialist
Lower anogenital screening and treatment
Addiction Medicine

While some of these fellowships are specific to Ob/Gyn and only accept those who completed Ob/Gyn residency, others exist within the broader fields of medicine or surgery. These fellowships provide valuable opportunities for networking outside of Ob/Gyn and can allow a graduate to become a bridge between fields.

How Do You Apply for and Choose a Nontraditional Fellowship Program?

Pursuing a nontraditional fellowship can often deviate from the classic application cycles listed by ABOG and the Electronic Residency Application Service®. Fellowship program websites will typically have the most important application information including eligibility requirements, deadlines, and a point of contact for questions. Generally, the application cycles will begin during the third year of residency. However, if a fourth-year resident decides to pursue a nontraditional fellowship, he/she/they should reach out to programs of interest, as there is always a possibility of unfilled spots or unaccredited positions. Practicing Ob/Gyns may also choose to pursue a nontraditional fellowship as their clinical interests develop beyond training.

Interviews may be conducted in-person or virtually. In addition to maintaining a well-rounded curriculum vitae, applicants should emphasize their interest in this specific field on their application and in their interviews. Fellowship training will reflect the practices and interests of the mentor faculty, so applicants should research what opportunities make a program unique when applying. Speaking with prior trainees is an excellent place to start.

There are several aspects to consider when searching for a nontraditional fellowship. While an Ob/Gyn residency or traditional fellowship has standards of competency as determined by ABOG, a nontraditional subspecialty fellowship often does not. Therefore, the clinical experiences and research opportunities of trainees will vary between institutions. The typical variables that are in line with what to consider when choosing a residency include geography and academic versus community settings. Furthermore, the location and training atmosphere can determine the patient populations and autonomy in training. When pursuing a nontraditional fellowship, it is also crucial to consider how Ob/Gyn training and the specialized fellowship training may complement each other. Joining a program that has subspecialists with a background in Ob/Gyn can help the trainee grow their skills obtained in residency and apply them to the subspecialty. Asking the program about their history of training fellows with a background in Ob/Gyn and reaching out to those prior fellows can be helpful.

Length of training can vary between fellowship programs even within the same nontraditional field. The most common example of this are programs that require an additional year of research. This additional time can be a great opportunity to become more established within a very small field, which in turn can help further networking, employment opportunities, and career trajectories.

From our experience, the most important factor to consider is mentorship. By aligning oneself with an accomplished member of the chosen field, a fellow will find more opportunities for productivity and networking. The professional connections and visibility built during fellowship will provide a direct pathway to jump starting a successful career in the chosen subspecialty. A way to gauge the quality of mentorship is to ask about fellow support to attend professional conferences, funding for research and publications, and learning about the career paths of prior fellows post graduation.

What Would Board Certification and My Career Following a Nontraditional Fellowship Look Like?

While pursuing a nontraditional fellowship, Ob/Gyn residency graduates are eligible to take the ABOG certifying exam. However, it is important to note that ABOG does not recognize nontraditional fellowships and, therefore, a board-eligible candidate must obtain unrestricted hospital privileges to perform Ob/Gyn in the form of moonlighting in order to collect cases. Familiarizing yourself with the ABOG Certifying Examinations eligibility and time requirements would be wise. Currently, physicians must achieve certification within eight years of the completion of their residency training. If eight years lapse, they must complete a minimum of six months of supervised practice in order to apply for the Qualifying or Certifying Examinations [1]. Many nontraditional fellowships have their own certifying examinations, allowing for dual board certification. Applicants should confirm that graduates are eligible for board certification if this is desired.

Completing a nontraditional fellowship is an excellent way to subspecialize your area of practice or expand your clinical capabilities. Many specialty-trained Ob/Gyns will devote a portion of their clinical time to run specialty clinics (i.e., disorders of sex development, vaginitis, sexual health) related to their nontraditional fellowship training and spend the remainder of their time practicing general Ob/Gyn. Others use their fellowship year(s) to begin a subspecialized career and go on to become subject matter experts. Whether you are considering a nontraditional fellowship in order to launch into another subspecialty or to further your generalist career, time in fellowship can yield exponential growth in your career.

Reference

1. *2024 Specialty Certifying Examination Bulletin*. American Board of Obstetrics and Gynecology. (2023, August). https://www.abog.org/specialty-certification/bulletins

Part II
Your First Job Search

Chapter 12
Where to Look for Jobs

Inara Omuso

Introduction

You are now in the driver's seat. Employers want you and, in the current state of healthcare, NEED you! For some of you, this may be your first real experience of applying for a career job, not just applying to continue your education and clinical experience. Take this opportunity to ask for what you want while highlighting your training, skills, and abilities. During your application process, also take time to highlight what you can bring to the practice while inquiring about what the practice can do to benefit you (i.e., your skills, your cases, work-life balance, change in environment, focused patient-population care, etc.).

Some practices are looking just to fill a position, and some are looking for a genuine member of a team; you can typically get a sense of which based on your interview (ask about physician turn-over, leadership opportunities, physician retention strategies, administrative duties)

Your first contract may be flawed, but avoid the major (and potentially expensive) pitfalls of malpractice, restrictive covenants, and exposure to case volume needed for your certification board exam. In this next section, we will review where to look for your next position. Subsequent chapters will provide an overview of the application process, address contractions and negotiations, and applying for hospital privileges and state licenses.

I. Omuso (✉)
Obstetrics and Gynecology, MedStar Medical Group, Clinton, MD, USA

A. Malik et al. (eds.), *An Obstetrician/Gynecologist's Path*,
https://doi.org/10.1007/978-3-031-87098-9_12

Where to Look

Where to look should begin with WHAT you are looking for. For many of you, this is your first full-time salaried career. You are now stepping out of the student-teacher role and into your full-fledged career. This is your opportunity to lay out your priorities and find a job that aligns with them. Remember, your first job out of residency does not have to be the perfect match; more than half of new residency graduates stay at their first job for only 2–3 years.

You are in the driver's seat more than at any other stage of your education and training.

In general, start your job search process 6–12 months in advance so that you can begin interviewing by the fall/winter of your fourth year.

What Are You Looking For

Again, your first job out of residency will likely not be your permanent career position; as your priorities change, the "what" in what you are looking for in your long-term career may also change. The vast majority of residents make changes in their career location and/or role within the first 3–5 years of their first job.

One thing to consider when looking is the type of practice you want to join.

(a) Academic-based positions: These positions are the ones you have been exposed to the most during residency, as these are the majority of your attendings. You are hired within a school or hospital residency program. The main benefits of these positions include access to teaching and administrative opportunities; they also tend to offer better benefits packages. Applying to your home institution also has its perks, as you know the system, the overall hospital/organization flow, and your future colleagues, and you tend to have a breadth of support during your transition from resident to attending.

(b) Private practice: These positions tend to be smaller than academic or hospital-employed groups as you are hired directly into another physician's business. These positions offer more autonomy and more opportunities for work-life balance, and they tend to provide higher base salaries. These roles can include office-only work but usually have a set call schedule, which can fluctuate based on the number of providers employed in the practice. Some private practices utilize OB hospitalists and locum tenens to reduce the potential call burden when the private practice call-to-provider ratio is too high.

(c) Hospital or health system employed: These positions could include a previously private practice subsequently absorbed into a healthcare system or private hospital. These positions tend to provide more resources (e.g., access to subspecialists), higher salaries, and bonus incentives.

(d) Hospitalists: These positions primarily cover hospital-based patient care (e.g., labor and delivery, OB triage/ED, floor consults, ER consults) and can also cover private providers' patients/deliveries. Some hospitalist positions also offer access to covering office patients in hospital-affiliated clinics. These positions allow for shift work while providing flexibility and control over your schedule.

(e) Locums tenens: This includes hospitalist-based work, but you are not hired by a specific hospital/practice; you serve as an independent contractor. These positions give you even more control over your schedule and provide more flexibility in location and duration of work.

Some other considerations when starting your application process:

- Where is your ideal location to practice?
- How far are you willing to commute?
- Is this a small, mid-sized, or large group practice?
- Are there opportunities for a partnership track?
- Are there research opportunities?
- Is there access to working with a Federally Qualified Health Center (FQHC)?
- What hospital support is offered: subspecialty support, closest tertiary care facility, level of NICU, in-house anesthesia, in-house operating team, emergency surgical services support, robotics training, outpatient surgery centers?
- What is the compensation model being used: RVU-based? Guaranteed salary? (This is reviewed in more detail in subsequent chapters.)
- Will you be covering multiple hospitals or offices? Is there hospital backup support? Additional night/weekend coverage? What is the anticipated call vs. office schedule?
- What is the standard vacation allotment, CME allotment, and maternity/paternity leave?

Where to Look

Once you get a sense of the type of position you are seeking, you can start using the following resources to find active positions available.

Your "home" institution (where you are completing your residency) is an excellent resource for networking. If you do not intend to stay on staff, you can ask the private groups that deliver or operate at your academic center about possible positions, in addition to asking your program director, prior resident graduates, or any of the other "off-site" physicians that you have been exposed to during residency.

If you have a specific area in mind, research the major hospitals or healthcare systems in that area and look at the groups with privileges there.

Career job boards offer a large database of available positions across the USA. These job boards are typically free, easily accessible, and provide exposure to large national healthcare groups, small private practices, academic positions, and non-academic groups.

The more common job boards include:

- ACOG Career Connect (online)
- ACOG Career Fair (virtual or in-person during the ACOG Annual Clinical & Scientific Meeting)
- Healthcare system websites: look for their physician posting sections
- Independent Hospitalist group websites—typically include full benefits like retirement packages, malpractice insurance, and CME allowance
- Locum tenens websites (more details below)

Recruiters typically reach out to you first and likely have already started if you are in your fourth year of residency. They can be a part of a private recruitment company, hired by a healthcare system, a locum tenens company, or a private group practice. If you decide to go this route, there is an abundance of recruiters for you to choose from, and you are not limited to only working with one at a time. Using a recruiter may also reduce the volume of individual searching you must do alone. Once you decide to use a recruiter, they usually start with an interview or survey to determine preferences and priorities and then present you with available opportunities. Remember who the recruiters have been hired by, as this may limit your offered positions. Also, inquire about any recruiter fees, as these may apply to you personally or be covered by the institution seeking employees.

Locum tenens positions are OKAY to apply to, even if you are coming straight out of residency.

These positions may be an opportunity for a "trial run" of a specific location, hospital system, or practice. When using a locum tenens company, make sure to inquire about:

- Malpractice insurance (a large portion of locum tenens do not offer this as a part of your contract)
- TERMINATION of contract requirements
- Their plan if the company dissolves during your active contract
- Number of jobs/positions available
- Telehealth options
- Any benefit packages (the vast majority do not offer these)
- Do they offer any travel and lodging allocation/reimbursement
- Remember your taxes (1099)! Consider paying quarterly, getting a dedicated accountant early for actual tax planning (consider starting an LLC)

If you want to pursue a locums position, look into opportunities for direct-employed internal locums/per diem positions. These positions usually provide a W-2 and additional healthcare benefits.

Plan to interview with multiple practices, even if you consider staying on staff at your residency program. However, you usually do not have to go on a similar interview odyssey as you did when applying for your residency position. Applying to a few positions may also give you leverage with negotiations along the way. And always remember that where you start your career does not have to be where you finish [1].

Reference

1. Heemstra J. 2020, October 12. The job market is tough. It's wise to explore different career options. Chemical & Engineering News. https://cen.acs.org/careers/employment/job-market-tough-s-wise/98/i39

Chapter 13
Applications

Inara Omuso

Job Applications

Most career connection and job search websites make it very easy to apply. You must create an account, upload your CV (with or without an official resume or cover letter), and submit these to your desired positions. Most recruiters will complete applications on your behalf after you submit your cover letter. In this section, we will review the basic components of a standard application.

Components of Your Application

Cover Letter

A cover letter is optional but allows you to individualize your requests to a specific position, outlining how the position potentially aligns with your desires for career development, teaching opportunities, etc., and also allows you a space to detail any of the specific skills that you are bringing to the position. Cover letters are also helpful for online applications.

Generally, a resume/CV portrays what you have done for your career development up to this point, and a cover letter highlights more of your future career goals [1].

General Structure

- Your information
- Their information

I. Omuso (✉)
Obstetrics and Gynecology, MedStar Medical Group, Clinton, MD, USA

A. Malik et al. (eds.), *An Obstetrician/Gynecologist's Path*,
https://doi.org/10.1007/978-3-031-87098-9_13

- Try to address the letter to a specific person
- Start with why you are interested and what experience you bring, then include 1–2 sentences about your background and other relevant experiences. Here are some tips:
  - Highlight specific skills and use positive descriptors (communication, service, leadership, teaching/education).
  - Mention whether you are looking for a position in that specific area, looking for research, and/or teaching opportunities.
- It should be about 250–500 words, less than one page.
- Consider making a short and long version depending on the application website, which may have limited characters.

Get feedback! From your attendings, residency program coordinators, recruiters, or family and acquaintances [1].

CV

Your CV (Curriculum Vitae, Latin for "course of life") highlights your academic history, professional history, and qualifications [2].

As the American College of Physicians explains, your CV should "[establish] a favorable image of your professionalism in the mind of the reader… [and also] emphasize your areas of strength and create an interest about you sufficient to result in a personal interview" (Borg, 2016).

Writing Your CV

Your CV should generally include your work experience, awards, scholarships or grants earned, coursework, research projects, and publications.

General template for your CV [3]:

1. Contact Information
2. Academic History
3. Professional experience, work experience, employment experience
4. Professional Affiliations and Honors
5. Publications, Presentations, and Other Activities
6. References

More detailed structure [2, 3]:

1. *Contact Information*
   (a) Full name, phone number, and email address (optional: add city, state, and ZIP)

(b) Designate current and permanent address

2. *Personal data* (marriage status, age) is OPTIONAL
3. *Academic history* (should be listed in reverse chronological order)

(a) List as institution, then dates; subtext should include the city and state (or country) and the degree obtained upon completion.

(i) Optional: for COLLEGE history, you can add your degree of focus and graduation titles, i.e., magna cum laude, etc.

(b) Avoid starting with institution abbreviations (this can be included in parentheses, especially if it is referenced elsewhere)
(c) Under RESIDENCY history

(i) Consider including a small section on what you did during your residency, for example:

1. "*Fulfilling the duties of an OB/GYN house staff member, including taking care of patients in the different subdivisions of the OB/GYN department for an underserved and urban population.*"
2. "*Participating in a resident-run, faculty-supervised community continuity clinic weekly.*"

(ii) Include administrative/academic chief roles

YOUR NAME, M.D/D.O/MBBS

Current Location | Phone Number | Email Address

EDUCATION

Residency Program (abbreviations as needed) **Dates(Month Year-Month Year)**
City, State
Obstetrics and Gynecology Resident
Academic chief resident

Institution (abbreviations as needed) **Dates**
City, State
Degree obtained

Example **Rutgers, The State University of New Jersey** **Sept 2006-May 2010**
New Brunswick, NJ
B.A, Psychology Major
Magna cum laude

Image (Created by Inara Omuso)

4. *Professional experience, work experience, employment experience*

(a) List by the organization, job title, and dates employed; start with your most recent job.
(b) Include the employer's name and address (can be city and state only).
(c) Designate full-time and part-time positions.
(d) Briefly list your job duties and experience gained (use action words).

(e) Avoid time gaps.
(f) *OPTIONAL: include significant duties, successes and achievements, research interests, committee assignments, etc.*
(g)

WORK EXPERIENCE

Company Name **Dates**
Location
Job Title
Brief overview of job duties and experience

Company Name **Dates**
Location
Job Title
Brief overview of job duties and experience

EXAMPLE **SMART (Science Medicine and Related Topics) Program** **June 2011-May 2012**
Newark, NJ
Lead Teacher (Summer 11th grade; Winter 11th/12th grade)
Summer SMART: included community service, in-class lectures on major community health issues, and advice on preparing for college
Winter SMART: lead teacher for 30-34 students during the weekend program. Prepared lesson plans and activities for students, including advice on pursuing a career in medicine

(h) Remember to KEEP IT UNIFORM and condensed.

Image (created by Inara Omuso)

5. *Licenses*: state-specific, dates issues, active status.
6. *Certifications*: it is okay to include certifications such as ACLS, BLS, NRP, USMLE, ABOG-board eligibility status or completion status.
7. *Professional associations*: include all ACTIVE memberships, significant appointments, and/or elections to positions or committees with dates; "significant activities completed under your leadership."
8. *Awards and honors*: keep descriptions brief and include dates; residency awards are outstanding to add here!
9. *Publications*:

   (a) Provide full bibliographic entries.
   (b) Clarify your role.
   (c) Include any or all of these examples:

      (i) Subheadings
      (ii) Presentations
      (iii) Invited lectures
      (iv) Abstracts
      (v) Books
      (vi) Chapter(s) in book
      (vii) Journal articles

10. *Research activities* (even if not completed to date)
11. *Community service*
12. *Grants and fellowships*
13. *Optional: Professional references, hobbies, and interests*

Once you have completed the writing process using the above template, have it proofread by family/friends/colleagues, a neutral hired party (ACOG Career Connect), or even your department chair. Remember to stay organized while applying to multiple practices [3].

References

1. Gallo A. How to write a cover letter. Harvard Business Review; 2024. https://hbr.org/2014/02/how-to-write-a-cover-letter
2. Indeed Editorial Team. 2024, April 9. How to write a CV: tips, template and example | *indeed.com*. How to write a CV: tips, template and example. https://www.indeed.com/career-advice/resumes-cover-letters/how-to-write-a-cv
3. Borg A. 2016, October 20. How to write a C.V.: tips for physicians and medical students. ACP: American College of Physicians. https://www.acponline.org/membership/medical-students/preparing-for-residency/how-to-write-a-cv-tips-for-physicians-and-medical-students

Chapter 14
The Interview Process

Carine-Ange Tagni

Introduction: "Setting the Stage for Success"

Welcome to the next chapter of your medical career! You've made it, and it's time to lock in that dream job. Having been on both sides of the interview table numerous times, I understand the uncertainty of whether the person across from you is the right fit. As an experienced Obstetrician/Gynecologist, I'm thrilled to guide you through the often-intimidating interview process for your first job. Throughout this chapter, we'll explore ten essential steps to help you master this process, ensuring you're well prepared and confident to seize the opportunities that come your way.

Step 1: "Charting Your Course—Define Your Preferences"

Before stepping into the interview room, you must map out your job preferences. By considering factors like the type of practice, setting, location, financial package, benefits, and practice philosophy, you create a roadmap for your career. Imagine yourself in different environments and consider what excites you the most. Let's take a closer look at each factor:

- *Financial Package*: What is your expected compensation, including salary, bonuses, and benefits?
- *Benefits*: What benefits are essential to your well-being and job satisfaction?
- *Location*: Where would you like to practice? Urban or rural? Near family or in a new city?

C.-A. Tagni (✉)
SiBelle Med Spa, Women's Health and Aesthetic, Horsham, PA, USA

A. Malik et al. (eds.), *An Obstetrician/Gynecologist's Path*,
https://doi.org/10.1007/978-3-031-87098-9_14

- *Type of Practice*: Do you envision yourself in an academic institution, a community-based practice, or a private clinic?
- *Setting*: Consider the environment that best aligns with your values and preferences.
- *Patient Load*: What patient load is ideal for you to balance your work and personal life?
- *Practice Philosophy*: Evaluate if the practice's approach aligns with your values and beliefs.

For example, if you're passionate about community-based women's health and a balanced lifestyle, your ideal position might be in a suburban private practice.

Step 2: "Dress to Impress—Scrubs Not Required"

We OBGYNs are known for our impeccable scrubs, but when it comes to interviews, the dress code is a bit different. Remember, your attire speaks volumes about your professionalism and attention to detail. Consider the following tips for dressing with impact:

- Opt for a well-fitting suit with a classic and professional style.
- Keep your accessories simple and elegant.
- Choose closed-toe shoes for a polished appearance.
- Dressing the part conveys your commitment and respect for the interview process, setting the stage for a successful encounter.

Step 3: "Immerse Yourself—Engage the Environment"

Your journey begins from the moment you walk into the practice. Engaging with the environment, from the office staff to the interviewer's office décor, is an essential part of making a positive impression. Here's how to immerse yourself:

- *Engage with Office Staff*: Approach office staff warmly and inquire about their experiences working at the practice. For example, ask, "What do you enjoy most about working here?" Building a rapport with the staff demonstrates your genuine interest and respect for the entire team.
- *Observe and Inquire*: Pay attention to details in the interviewer's office, such as honors, plaques, and photographs. Ask about the items that pique your interest, as this demonstrates your curiosity and engagement. For instance, if you notice a prestigious award, you can ask, "I noticed the award on your shelf. Can you tell me more about it and its significance for the practice?"

Engaging with the environment builds a positive rapport, showcasing your interest and making the interview more comfortable for both parties.

Step 4: "Asking the Right Questions—Yes, They're Watching"

A prepared candidate is an impressive candidate. Jot down questions based on your preferences, as they'll demonstrate your seriousness and engagement. Think of these questions as your navigation tools, steering the conversation in a direction that helps you better understand the potential role. Here are some examples:

- *Financial Package*: "Could you provide details about the compensation structure, including the base salary, bonuses, and benefits?"
- *Benefits*: "What benefits are offered, and how do they contribute to the overall compensation package?"
- *Location*: "Can you describe the community and the lifestyle it offers for physicians?"
- *Type of Practice*: "What is the practice's mission and vision, and how does it align with the care I want to provide?"
- *Setting*: "Tell me more about the clinic or hospital setting and how it complements the practice's goals."
- *Patient Load*: "What is the typical patient load, and how does the practice ensure a manageable workload for its physicians?"
- *Practice Philosophy*: "How does the practice's philosophy impact the approach to patient care?"

These questions serve as your compass, guiding the interview toward a mutual understanding of whether the opportunity aligns with your expectations.

Step 5: "Elevator Pitch—Not Just for Elevators"

Every OBGYN has a unique story that sets them apart. During the interview, emphasize what makes you stand out and share your passion for the field. Here are some examples of how you can underline your uniqueness:

- *Share a Personal Story*: You could share a personal story of a memorable case that ignited your passion for OBGYN. For instance, "I'll never forget the time I was part of a high-risk pregnancy case where our team's dedication helped save both the mother and baby."
- *Highlight Unique Qualities*: Discuss unique qualities or skills that you possess. For example, if you have proficiency in a specialized technique, such as minimally invasive surgery, emphasize how this skill can benefit the practice and its patients.

Emphasizing your uniqueness is your chance to shine right from the start.

Step 6: "The Balancing Act—Include Your Spouse"

If you're married, consider including your spouse in the interview process. A happy home life can significantly influence your career satisfaction, making it essential to ensure your spouse is comfortable with the practice and the location. Here's how to approach this:

- *Request to Include Your Spouse*: It's always a good idea to inquire if you can bring your spouse along on an interview trip. The practice's willingness to accommodate this request indicates their support for work-life balance.
- *Meet Employees and Partners*: When you bring your spouse, request introductions to employees and partners at the practice. This allows your spouse to get a feel for the environment and the people they'll be interacting with if you accept the position.
- *Explore the Community*: Let your spouse explore the community to get a sense of where you might be living. It's important for both of you to feel comfortable with the location.

For example, you can express your intention to include your spouse and ask, "We value a supportive community. Can you provide more information about the work-life balance and the community here?"

Step 7: "Maintain Professionalism—Keep It Honest"

Honesty is the cornerstone of professionalism during an interview. It's important to be candid while framing potentially challenging aspects of your career in a positive light. To maintain professionalism:

- *Frame Challenges Positively*: If you need to discuss a less favorable aspect of your career, focus on how it contributed to your professional growth. For instance, you can say, "I faced a particularly challenging case that taught me the value of resilience and collaboration."
- *Refrain from Negative Remarks*: Resist the temptation to speak negatively about previous employers or colleagues. Be intentional about maintaining a positive and professional demeanor throughout the interview.

Honesty and professionalism are highly valued during the interview process.

Step 8: "Concise Clarity—Keep Answers to the Point"

During the interview, it's crucial to provide concise but comprehensive answers. Let's explore how you can effectively communicate during the interview:

- *Clarity and Conciseness*: Ensure that your answers are clear and concise. Avoid unnecessary elaboration while making sure your responses are thorough.
- *Honesty in Uncertainty*: If you don't know the answer to a question, don't hesitate to admit it. It's better to be honest about your limitations. For example, you can say, "I'm not familiar with that particular procedure, but I'm eager to learn and contribute to the practice in any way I can."

The interview can highlight your proficiency in effectively communicating complex medical information to patients and colleagues.

Step 9: "Relationship First—Delay Contract Negotiations"

While the initial interview is a critical step in the process, there is a better time for contract negotiations. It's essential to focus on evaluating potential working relationships with employers. Here's how to approach this:

- *Focus on Relationship-Building*: Concentrate on getting to know the practice and the team, understanding their culture and values, and allowing them to get to know you.
- *Save Contract Details*: Delay discussions about contract specifics for a later stage when both parties are confident that it's a good fit. This approach allows you to establish a solid foundation for your working relationship.

Building a solid working relationship is essential before delving into contractual negotiations.

Step 10: "Closing the Bag—The Art of the Farewell"

After the interview, make a point to express your gratitude and continue the dialogue. Here's how to wrap up the interview process effectively:

- *Express Gratitude in Person*: Take a moment to express your gratitude to the interviewer and the practice's team. A sincere thank you is always appreciated.
- *Obtain a Business Card*: Request a business card from your contact at the practice. This card will be instrumental for sending a personalized thank-you note, a thoughtful gesture that leaves a lasting positive impression.
- *Send a Thank-You Note*: Send a personalized thank-you note within a reasonable timeframe. Express your continued interest in the position and enthusiasm to join the team.

Capping Off the Essentials: "Preparing for the Future"

As you transition from your OBGYN residency to the next phase of your career as an attending physician, there are additional elements that can contribute to your interview success in securing your first job. Learning from real-life examples, whether shared by seasoned OBGYNs, colleagues who have recently made the transition, or your own experiences during residency, can provide invaluable practical insights and inspiration as you embark on this exciting journey. In addition, researching salary ranges, patient demographics, and practice trends in your desired location and setting will empower you to negotiate compensation and evaluate the compatibility of prospective positions with your career goals. Whether you are considering academic institutions, community-based practices, private clinics, or even locum tenens opportunities, adapting your strategy to each setting will be essential for your success.

Stay informed! Evolving healthcare regulations, the impact of telemedicine, changing patient demographics, and other factors will undoubtedly shape the landscape of your practice. Being aware of these challenges and trends will not only help you navigate them successfully but also position you as a forward-thinking and adaptable physician.

Finally, as you prepare for interviews and the next career phase, understand the importance of cultural sensitivity and diversity. Demonstrating your commitment to providing inclusive and patient-centered care by navigating these aspects respectfully will set you apart as a compassionate and culturally aware OBGYN.

Conclusion: "Your Journey Begins Here"

In the ever-transforming landscape of Obstetrics and Gynecology, the interview process is your gateway to success. Be sure to ask the right questions and explore every aspect of the job to ensure it aligns with your goals. The journey may be challenging, but with these steps, you're well prepared to embark on a rewarding path in this field. Always remember, you are an exceptional OBGYN! Good luck on your path to a fulfilling career in this field.

Chapter 15
Contracts and Negotiations

Inara Omuso

Letter of Intent

After completing your interview process, some practices will provide a letter of intent before offering a detailed contract. This letter of intent should clearly state the anticipated salary and term of the future contract. It can also detail any sign-on bonuses, including moving expenses.

This letter is not always offered; you may be offered a contract directly. You must clarify with the potential future employee a timeline for you to review and sign the letter of intent or contract. Even the letter of intent can be negotiated, so it should not deter you from signing before accepting the final contract and start date.

Basics of a Contract

Give yourself time to review the contract with an attorney and/or family/friends. Almost all contracts allow some negotiation, so do not hesitate to make requests. The following sections include the core components that should be included in an offered contract.

Work Details (Schedule, Location)

Your contract should clearly detail your anticipated job responsibilities, including weekly hours, days in the office, average patient volume, and shifts per week/month.

I. Omuso (✉)
Obstetrics and Gynecology, MedStar Medical Group, Clinton, Southern Maryland, MD, USA

A. Malik et al. (eds.), *An Obstetrician/Gynecologist's Path*,
https://doi.org/10.1007/978-3-031-87098-9_15

It should include details about the model used for reimbursement of work done beyond baseline requirements (i.e., extra shifts in a month, RVUs beyond expected, tier systems).

Look for specific definitions of your anticipated practice location(s). Contracts are not required to include practice locations beyond your anticipated primary location, but they should give some verbiage related to expectations beyond the primary location. *Negotiation tip: If any new locations are added after you sign, consider requesting more details be added to the contract regarding anticipated schedule changes.*

Look for employer-based definitions of FTE—full-time equivalent, 40-hour workweek.

Interview point: review details about how the call schedule is divided and whether it depends on the number of FTEs. Do they use locums to assist with the weekend calls?

Look for a section that details any specific restrictions on work outside of your primary employer, such as FQHC clinics, working with Planned Parenthood, or locums/moonlighting. *Negotiation tip: if you are joining an academic-based practice, inquire about allotted time for specific administrative/academic responsibilities as well as potential allocated for research opportunities*

Compensation Model

The anticipated compensation model should be clear within your contract. Generally, most practices follow either a fixed or variable compensation model, a combination of both or transition from a fixed model to a productivity model after a set amount of time. Most academic, health system, and hospital-employed practices use a work relative value units (wRVU) model (that typically begins with a guaranteed salary). Some private practices use a collections-based compensation model. Locum and hospitalist positions tend to be based more on shift- and time-based compensation models [1]. Regardless, your contract should clearly state how your compensation is calculated and specifically detail the time frame for any transition away from the base salary.

As stated before, most practices follow a fixed or variable compensation model. A fixed compensation model offers you a guaranteed base salary independent of your productivity and overall performance. This should be detailed in your salary as either a yearly sum or an hourly rate. Even with fixed compensation, your contract should still have room for the evolution of your salary/compensation over time.

A variable compensation model allows your salary to depend on multiple modalities based on productivity and performance. Productivity is generally calculated by work relative value units (wRVU), which are values set by the Centers for Medicare & Medicaid Services (CMS) for clinical activities spanning the office, hospital, and operating room. Your contract should specifically state the role of RVUs in calculating your salary, whether they equate to your total salary or provide a production-based bonus ABOVE your base salary. The contract can also detail the conversion factor used to determine the pay per RVU [2]. Some practices use a tiered approach to the productivity model, allowing you to see what your RVU goal is to meet your baseline salary and the RVU goal to receive a bonus above this; this, too, should be specifically detailed in the contract.

Negotiation tip: it is important to determine how your RVUs are tracked and the frequency at which your RVU report will be reviewed with you. It is best to establish some form of review (meeting, generated report) monthly, especially if your total salary is dependent on your RVUs

Interview tip: inquire about how many providers exceed their RVU threshold annually

Another compensation model that has been used more frequently in private practice is a salary based on collections or what you, as an individual provider, generate for the practice. Again, this should be clearly stated within the contract.

Clarity on how post-termination compensation will be handled should exist within the compensation portion of the contract and/or the termination of the contract term.

Restrictive Covenant

As of April 23, 2024, the Federal Trades Commission has issued a final rule banning non-competes nationwide. Specifically, the FTC stated that "[the non-compete] is an unfair method of competition—and therefore a violation of section 5—for persons to, among other things, enter into non-compete clauses ("non-competes") with workers on or after the final rule's effective date" [3]. This ruling came into effect in late August 2024. This ban was initially proposed in January 2024 and strongly backed by the American Medical Association (AMA) [4]. Before this ruling, non-compete bans varied by state. Non-competes allowed employers to define a small or large radius within which you could not practice upon terminating your contract. The radius and timeframe of the non compete would vary by location and practice. It was important that aspects of the contract clearly state the primary location of your non-compete, as multiple-office practices could cumulate in a very large non-compete radius. Some non-competes, especially in densely populated areas, could last 12–36 months. Other restrictive covenants would allow flexibility of the non-compete to refer to full scope or practice or allow for laborist-/hospitalist-only work within the non-compete radius [2].

Malpractice

As OB/GYNs, we work in an extremely high liability profession. Your contract must include how your malpractice insurance is covered by the employer. Some states provide malpractice coverage, but many providers must also have a private policy. The main types of malpractice policies follow either claims-based or occurrence-based coverage; please refer to the detailed Chap. 17 for more information.

Regardless of which type of malpractice policy your employer offers, it is important that you get a copy of your insurance policy, its terms, the related contact information for the policy carrier, and details related to any claims made. This policy information should be requested from your residency program and is generally needed when applying for hospital privileges.

Term and Termination

Another key component of your contract is the term and details related to termination. This should be clearly laid out in any contract that you sign.

The signing term of your contract can range from 1 to 3 years and can be linked to other components of your contract, such as your base salary, after which you must follow a productivity-based compensation model. The termination of the contract should relay the following information:

- Termination of contract without cause for both the employer and the provider
- Termination of contract with cause, including immediate termination
- Disability clause
- Unexpected death clause

Termination of contract without cause can be restrictive within the first few years of your signing, ranging from 30 to 180 days. In general, this tends to be the more accurate "term" of your contract as it is the guaranteed time that the details within your contract can be upheld. Most academic/hospital-employed/healthcare system-employed contracts range from 60 to 90 days and should have the same time frame for the employee and the provider to submit notice of termination. *Contract red flag: a large discrepancy between the allotted time for the employee to give notice* vs. *the provider or termination of contract less than 60 days for non-locums or hospitalist positions.* Some employees offer only a minimum-term length for the first 1–3 years of your contract and thus may not allow without cause termination of the contract.

Terms of immediate termination are typically related to disciplinary actions from medical boards, hospital boards, or directly from CMS. Some practice-specific terms of immediate termination may include significant delays in medical records, non-adherence to certain practice or hospital policies, or persistent grievances from patients, colleagues, and/or clinical staff members.

As a reminder, most disability terms should include the consecutive days of disability count and ideally match your existing disability insurance policy.

Lastly, your employer should include details related to payment of bonuses after notice of contract termination (especially sign-on bonuses) and RVUs (what you were reimbursed vs what you actually earned). These payments may be removed from your paychecks in the last few months, so plan accordingly!

Benefits

Your offered benefits may not be comprehensively outlined in your contract. The main components of your related benefits that should be included are paid time off, partner-buy-in opportunities, incentive pay, CME allocations, expectations for non-clinical responsibilities (attendance at department meetings, board certification requirements, maintenance of board certification requirements), and other related benefits.

The following may or may not be included in your written contract but are among the standard offered benefits for non-locum positions.

- Health and life insurance: inquire if this is offered for just you or your whole family
- Disability insurance

Retirement insurance: Inquire about when you qualify for matching; also, be aware that not all retirement policies automatically come into effect. There is no need to lose a year's worth of savings!

- Moving expenses
- Sign-on bonus: again, inquire about how this will be repaid in the event of early termination
- Incentive pay
- Retention bonus, value, and quality bonuses
- CME: travel, conferences, speeches
- Boards, certifications, memberships, licensure coverage/reimbursement
- Maternity/paternity leave
- Student loan forgiveness: Public Service Loan Forgiveness, direct pay from practice, state-based allocated funds
- Travel expenses (especially if a multi-office/hospital practice)

Negotiations

The main goals of your contract negotiation are to set clear expectations, advocate for yourself, your skills, and your work-life balance, and ensure that what is being offered is competitive for the area/region. Before your negotiation, your contract should have been reviewed by at least a contract attorney; depending on the time-frame you are working with, consider also having it reviewed by a trusted attending, mentor, or family/friend.

Remember that you are now stepping out of the strict mentor/student role of a resident and into a colleague/partner or mentor/colleague role, so do not hesitate to ask for what you want.

To ensure that you are being offered a competitive salary, briefly review the Medical Group Management Association (MGMA) annual report on comparative compensation data per specialty and region. You can address these points when speaking to your potential employer by asking how they keep up with competitive market value and how they balance pay, benefits, and growth opportunities.

Take the time to circle back to the "what are you looking for" when you first began your job search, as certain contract components will carry more weight.

Look out for these RED FLAGS!

- Unclear compensation model
- Unclear working duties
- Unclear restrictive covenant
- Pressure to sign a contract within a short period of time
- Issues with the termination of the agreement (for non-locums <60 days)
- Vague malpractice policies
- Unclear or vague causes for dismissal/termination

Though signing a contract is time-sensitive, you must exercise due diligence and have it reviewed before signing!

References

1. Hudgins A. Factors to consider before signing a physician contract. Health eCareers. https://www.healthecareers.com/career-resources/salary-and-benefits/8-factors-to-consider-before-signing-a-contract. 26 Oct 2023.
2. Sarnoski K. 5 key differences of various practice types – physician contract reviews: contract diagnostics. Physician Contract Reviews | Contract Diagnostics. https://contractdiagnostics.com/blog/5-key-differences-of-various-practice-types/. 28 Mar 2023.
3. Non-Compete Clause Rule. 2024.
4. Adriatico A. FTC announces rule Banning noncompetes. Human Resources Director – US. https://www.ftc.gov/news-events/news/press-releases/2024/04/ftc-announces-rule-banning-noncompetes. 24 Apr 2024.

Chapter 16
Applying for Privileges and License

Inara Omuso

Applying for your state medical license and hospital privileges can be quite tedious. Some states are faster and more straightforward than others regarding your state medical license. Most hospitals use their own delineation of privileges application, which typically does not translate to other hospitals and must be renewed annually.

Key points when applying for your license and hospital privileges: stay organized, stay connected, and stay up to date.

Stay Organized Many credentialing systems can be complex and sometimes seem repetitive; organizing your most commonly requested documents in a singular area is best. You should also keep a short list of prior claims and pending cases available, as these are typically requested during your hospital credentialing application.

Stay Connected You will need references whenever you apply for new privileges. At the minimum, it is required to have a professional reference, but some hospitals require a reference from a prior department chair or lead physician at your prior practice. If you are coming directly from residency, ask your attendings and department chair early, as this tends to be the rate-limiting step in the application process. Although most people do not stay at their first job, it is still important to attempt to make some professional connections that can serve as a reference for your future hospital privileges application. It is also best practice to use references you have worked with, ideally within the last 5 years.

Maintaining your residency administrator, office manager, and medical staff office contact is also beneficial. They can more readily provide you with certain credentials, certificates, vaccination status, prior training, and your very important case logs!

I. Omuso (✉)
Obstetrics and Gynecology, MedStar Medical Group, Clinton, Southern Maryland, MD, USA

A. Malik et al. (eds.), *An Obstetrician/Gynecologist's Path*,
https://doi.org/10.1007/978-3-031-87098-9_16

Negotiation tip: applying for your state medical license and privileges applications can quickly add up; requesting that your future employer cover or reimburse these costs is very reasonable.

Stay Up to Date Keep an up-to-date record of your vaccinations, BLS/ACLS/PALS training (try to get this updated within your 4th year of residency), EFM certification, DEA, CDS, and ABOG/ACOG membership. Keep a log of the OB/GYN/office cases that you do; your residency program's medical staff office will aid with this, and your future practice should as well. When it comes to delineating privileges (the procedures and surgeries you desire to do at the hospital), your application will inquire about the volume of requested privileges you have done in a designated time frame. Delineation of privileges ranges from admitting a patient to doing a sacrocolpoplexy. Some hospitals still require certain cases to be proctored for a set amount of cases before you can complete them on your own.

As an overview, here is a basic checklist of the most common requests when applying for new hospital privileges

- Prior claims
- Professional references
- Specific start and end dates of prior practice
- Major cases, robotics cases, or other specialty surgical cases
- Prior leadership roles
- Prior office manager contact information

Negotiation tip: Inquire if your future employer has clinical (or non-clinical) staff who assist with maintaining up-to-date privileges, credentialing, and certifications by tracking renewal dates; this is a major help if available!

Chapter 17
Malpractice

Robin Perry

For those of us with careers in Obstetrics and Gynecology, dealing with medical malpractice is initially quite overwhelming. Yet over the course of time, dealing with malpractice becomes less of a "trauma" and more of a "cost of doing business" in medicine. Like any other aspect of business management, we need to become familiar with the concepts surrounding medical negligence and to make intelligent decisions around the prevention and management of a malpractice claim. As we make the transition from trainee to independent practitioner, we also transition from the role of supporting team member to that of medical staff member who is fully accountable for the quality of care provided. This transition has implications for medical malpractice and is particularly significant for obstetrician gynecologists. According to the Medscape Malpractice Report 2021, 79% of the Obstetrician Gynecologists who responded reported that they have been named in a malpractice suit [1]. Given this level of occurrence, being educated and prepared regarding the impact of malpractice on you as a provider is, in my opinion, essential for job satisfaction and wellness for the Obstetrician Gynecologist.

Definitions

Let us review some basic facts. In the US legal system, malpractice is considered a tort. A tort is a wrongful act, other than a breach of contract, for which relief may be obtained in the form of damages (a financial payout) or an injunction (a court

R. Perry (✉)
Division of Maternal-Fetal Medicine, Department of Obstetrics and Gynecology,
Cooper Medical School of Rowan University and Cooper University Health Care,
Camden, NJ, USA

A. Malik et al. (eds.), *An Obstetrician/Gynecologist's Path*,
https://doi.org/10.1007/978-3-031-87098-9_17

ordered act). Medical malpractice is an act or continuing conduct of a professional, which does not meet the standard of professional competence, and results in provable damages to his/her client or patient. Therefore, malpractice has three components and all three must be present to prove malpractice: (1) deviation from the standard of care, (2) a proven damage, and (3) the deviation must be shown to have caused the damage. When all three components are present, malpractice has occurred. You might wonder how the "standard of care" can be defined. In medical malpractice cases, the basic concept is that standard of care is based on the customary practices of the average provider. In other words, the healthcare provider's patient care is judged based on what a reasonably competent provider with the same level of training would do. In the end, expert witnesses provide testimony regarding the standard of care and if it was met. It is important to remember that, in the United States, we have malpractice laws to allow for financial restitution when an individual has been harmed by another individual's negligence or error. Not all harm is caused by negligence, but when it is, the individual harmed can pursue a malpractice claim as recourse.

Malpractice Insurance

Everyone can make mistakes, even highly trained professionals. Since mistakes in medicine can lead to a malpractice claim, how can a physician protect themselves? On a very practical level, obtaining medical malpractice insurance will help to protect our personal assets. If a monetary judgment is awarded, the insurance company will cover the expense. When looking for a new position, it is critical to understand the importance of, and necessity for, malpractice insurance and the types of policies available. The first question you need to answer is, should I buy a malpractice policy or can I go without insurance (often termed going bare)? There are seven states in the United States where malpractice insurance is mandated: Colorado, Connecticut, Kansas, Massachusetts, New Jersey, Rhode Island, and Wisconsin. In these states, going bare is not an option. ACOG provides a great review on what questions you might ask if considering going bare.

Most Obstetrician Gynecologists do purchase, or their employers provide, medical malpractice insurance. To better understand the type of coverage you might be offered, let's review some definitions. There are two common types of medical professional liability insurance available—"occurrence" and "claims-made" coverage.

An occurrence policy will cover a claim for an incident that happened while the policy was in effect, even if the claim is filed after the policy is terminated. Many obstetricians prefer this type of coverage because claims for impaired infants can occur years after birth. Occurrence coverage is usually more expensive and may be more difficult to find.

A claims-made policy, in comparison, will cover you for claims only if the following two conditions are met: (1) the claim must be reported during the period the policy was in effect and (2) the claim must be a result of an incident that occurred when the policy was in effect. This type of policy will not cover claims filed after the policy is no longer in effect, even though the incident occurred while the policy was in effect. These types of policies tend to be less expensive and, therefore, more easily afforded. There is a reason for the savings.

Consider this example—say you have been offered a dream job right out of residency, with a great salary in a great location and the practice offers you a claims-made policy for malpractice coverage, from Insurance Company A. They explain that this is the type of coverage all the physicians in the practice have. It will cover you for $1 million per case and $3 million per year, meeting the requirements of the medical staff office in your hospital. Five years later your spouse gets transferred to a new city, you inform your practice that you need to relocate and begin your job search. You find a wonderful job in the new city and offer your official letter of resignation. On the date that your resignation occurs your claims made policy ends. *Unless you want to personally continue to pay your insurance premiums to Insurance Company A, which can be quite expensive, you will most likely discontinue your policy.* Your new job offers you Occurrence Coverage from Insurance Company B. You will be covered for any event that occurs while you have this coverage, independent of when a suit occurs. You are very happy about your new job and your insurance coverage.

You do, however, still have a problem. After you switch insurance plans, you no longer have coverage for future claims, within the statute of limitations, on incidents from the previous five years. The statute of limitations, or time allowed for someone to file a claim after an incident, varies by state. In the case of newborns, the statute of limitations often ends after the age of majority, which in most states is 18 years. So, in our example, as an obstetrician gynecologist you are personally at risk for any malpractice claim that might occur secondary to birth outcomes for quite a number of years after you terminate your claims made policy.

Luckily, you do have a choice at this time. You can either take your chances and go bare or you can attempt to access continuing insurance coverage for that time period. The most common approach to obtaining coverage in this setting is to purchase tail coverage. Tail coverage protects you when a claim (related to an incident that happened while you were insured under a claims-made policy) is filed after that policy is no longer in effect. The cost of tail coverage can vary from two to ten times the cost of your last annual premium and will vary based on years of practice and claims history. Going back to our example, in order to take that great new position, you would need to finance a significant additional expense, often in excess of one hundred thousand dollars. Adding this expense to your relocation budget can be quite overwhelming. Fortunately, in your new role, you have been offered occurrence coverage, which will assure that you will not have this stress should you need to leave your new job in the future.

In addition to having an appropriate malpractice policy, it is advisable to be aware of malpractice risk and how you can minimize that risk. Providing evidence-based care is at the cornerstone of risk management strategies for a practitioner. Accurately documenting that care, as well as the reasoning behind your management decisions, can keep you from being named in a case. One of the things I like to ask myself to assure that my documentation is adequate is, "If this case has an unexpected poor outcome, does my documentation support that my actions were necessary and appropriate?" The best way to manage your risk is to avoid being named in a case in the first place.

Taking the time to have thorough, meaningful informed consent discussions with your patients is also fundamental in any strategy to reduce medical professional liability risk. The requirements for informed consent vary greatly state by state. In general, patients need to know their medical condition, the treatment being recommended, likely benefits of the treatment, relative probability of success, risk and complications that could be involved, alternative treatments along with their risks and benefits, and possible consequences of not being treated. Obtaining informed consent is not just for major surgeries or procedures but also applies to recommending office procedures, ordering diagnostic tests, and prescribing medications. Documenting this discussion including the patient's questions and how they were answered can be critical in avoiding a malpractice suit. The use of clear communication and shared decision-making will significantly aid in malpractice risk mitigation.

The use of electronic health records (EHR) has added a new dimension to documentation risk management. The use of the cut and paste function may make your documentation faster, but is easily apparent in a medicolegal review and can introduce outdated information, replicate incorrect information, result in unnecessarily lengthy notes, and at times misrepresent the level of care provided. All medical documentation must reflect what is happening with the individual patient at the time the note is written. While templates can be timesaving, we must modify the template as needed to reflect the care we provide to each individual patient. Keep in mind that the EHR automatically records the users name, timestamps when you open your note and when you close or sign the note, and if copy/paste has been used, where you copied from and who authored that document. Also, remember that our notes are not only reviewed by colleagues for medical practice, coders for billing, and attorneys for litigation but also by our patients who have full access to their medical records in a much more immediate fashion than ever before. We need to use great care in how we utilize this powerful tool.

One final strategy to minimize malpractice risk is to be familiar with what to do when an adverse event occurs. Adverse events are at times preventable and other times not. They often significantly impact the patient and their family as well as the providers involved. After an adverse outcome, patients expect and want timely and full disclosure of the event, an acknowledgment of responsibility, an understanding of what happened, expressions of sympathy, and a discussion of what will be done to prevent recurrence. Accomplishing all of this is not easy. Adverse events are often traumatic to the providers, who are then responsible for disclosure and documentation of the event. In your role as an attending physician, you need to know who in your practice or healthcare system you need to inform of an adverse event. This is usually your malpractice carrier or your risk management team. You should be aware of who you can contact to help you manage and disclose the adverse event, this may be a mentor or a more experienced physician. It is often helpful to have the disclosure discussion with someone who has done it before, a more experienced individual who feels comfortable with this type of difficult conversation. Accurate documentation of the discussion is also important. For more information on adverse event disclosure, see ACOG Committee Opinion #681 [2].

Even after many years of training and experience, mistakes can be made and adverse outcomes can occur even with appropriate high-quality care. Either of these scenarios can lead to a claim being filed and we need to be prepared for that. Having appropriate malpractice insurance, staying current on evidence-based practice, obtaining appropriate informed consent, openly and compassionately communicating with patients particularly when a mistake is made or an adverse outcome occurs, and quality documentation will all help to protect you if a claim is made against you. When it comes to navigating medical malpractice issues in obstetrics and gynecology, being forewarned is being forearmed.

References

1. Gallegos A. Medscape malpractice report 2021. 19 Nov 2021. https://www.medscape.com/slideshow/2021-malpractice-report-6014604port2021.
2. Committee Opinion No. 681: disclosure and discussion of adverse events. Obstet Gynecol. 2016;128(6):e257–e261. https://doi.org/10.1097/AOG.0000000000001816.
3. https://www.acog.org/practice-management/professional-liability.

Chapter 18
Practicing Academic Medicine

Elizabeth A. Gagliardi

What is academic medicine? Academic medicine is a generalized term for a setting where physicians may practice clinical medicine while also having the opportunity to perform research and train new and future physicians (fellows, residents, medical students). Positions in academic medicine come in many different forms, with some physicians focusing solely on training and others solely on research, but most positions in academic medicine incorporate a ratio of clinical practice, education, and research. Traditionally, academic medicine occurs in large, tertiary care centers associated with medical schools and research funding, but it can also be practiced in smaller, community hospitals. Most academicians teach across all stages of learning (medical students through fellows), but a physician in academics can focus their teaching on a subset of learners, as well. In summary, academic medicine can occur in any setting where there are learners.

Physicians working in academics usually have an academic appointment at a medical school, or at the very least an association with a medical school. Physicians who work in academic centers (larger tertiary care centers affiliated with medical schools) often integrate teaching into all their job responsibilities: they precept medical students and residents in clinic; teach learners on labor and delivery, the OR and the inpatient floors; and incorporate and mentor learners through their research. In a tertiary care center, teaching and mentoring occur on inpatient units, in outpatient clinics, in labs, and online. However, academic medicine can also take the form of a medical student shadowing a physician in their private practice clinic. For those hoping to participate in academic medicine, there are many different ways to be involved and to teach.

E. A. Gagliardi (✉)
Division of Gynecology, Lahey Hospital and Medical Center, Burlington, MA, USA

Department of Obstetrics, Gynecology and Reproductive Biology at Harvard Medical School, Boston, MA, USA

A. Malik et al. (eds.), *An Obstetrician/Gynecologist's Path*,
https://doi.org/10.1007/978-3-031-87098-9_18

The benefits of academic medicine primarily stem from involvement in education. Physicians who teach often state that their involvement with learners reminds them of their own excitement and awe as a learner and re-invigorates them when the practice of medicine becomes more routine. Teaching requires that you stay current with evolving data and research and that you practice evidence-based medicine. I often find that my students and residents teach me as much as I teach them. They are constantly reading and inquiring why medicine is practiced in one way rather than another. In the operating room and on the labor floor, the process of explaining why we approach patient care in a certain way (for instance why we would use a 5 mm port versus an 8 mm one in a laparoscopic case) helps the attending to think through their own approaches to patient care and then refine them, if indicated. For those participating in academic communities, there are educational resources for the attendings themselves, such as Grand Rounds and educational lectures/webinars, to help the faculty keep current with advances in OB/Gyn and associated fields.

In academic centers, education and research are often compensated with time, and sometimes also with money. Attendings in academic centers usually have time built into their day-to-day schedules to spend on academic pursuits. Depending on their roles, a percentage of their time is dedicated to education of learners. The common term surrounding time in academic practice is full time equivalents (FTEs). A physician who works full time is a 1.0 FTE while a physician who works 80% of the time is a 0.8 FTE (this presumes a forty hour work week, which is often a false premise as most full-time clinicians work more than this). FTE can further be divided into clinical, research, academic, and administrative time. A physician who works full-time (1.0 FTE) who sees patients four days a week (clinic/L and D/OR) but spends one day a week doing research would be 0.8 FTE clinical and 0.2 FTE research. A residency program director who sees patients three days a week and runs the residency two days a week would be 0.6 FTE clinical and 0.4 FTE administrative. Most academic attendings will have some academic/teaching time built into their FTE (usually 0.1 or 0.2 FTE, which amounts to a half or full day a week) to allow them time to address their academic endeavors (i.e., create lectures, meet with learners to give feedback, precept learners in the simulation lab, etc.). In addition to this protected time, attending physicians in leadership roles may also be paid a separate stipend.

Attending physicians working in academic centers are often appointed to the faculty of the medical school associated with the center. Faculty appointments are included as part of job contracts and new attending physicians generally start as instructors. As a physician's career develops and the attending obtains grants, publishes research, develops into leadership roles, and creates clinical innovation, they may apply for promotion within the faculty with the subsequent levels after Instructor being Assistant Professor, then Associate Professor, then Professor. Each subsequent faculty level is considered more prestigious. It is rare for clinical faculty to be appointed to tenure track, but promotions can be tied to stipends and vacation time by the department (for instance, $10,000 raise with each promotion and an additional 5 days of vacation). The benefits of faculty appointment also include faculty development programming, funding opportunities, professional awards, access to library resources/journals, membership in research databases, and eligibility for educator discounts.

While academic medicine may be attractive to some, there are also potential downsides. For those in private practice who teach, there is usually a small stipend, but this often does not compensate for the decreased revenue from seeing less patients to allow time to teach. For those practicing in academic centers, the disadvantages can be even greater. Salaries in academic centers are generally much lower than those of private practice practitioners or those practicing in multi-specialty groups. Academic centers often use non-financial incentives to attract physicians, such as protected academic time or prestige of faculty appointment. But, non-academic jobs have more flexibility to provide financial incentives like signing bonuses or productivity bonuses. Even in academic centers where productivity bonuses are offered, the volume of patients that can be treated is decreased due to the extra time it takes to teach/mentor students; this applies to labor and delivery, operating rooms, and outpatient clinics. While faculty appointments might be prestigious, the promotion process is extremely complex and technical, requiring multiple milestones to be met in multiple areas, and the financial rewards of promotion tend to be quite limited. In addition, many new attendings struggle to balance the opposing goals of teaching and promoting learner autonomy while developing their own confidence and autonomy. For a new attending physician, it can be difficult to master the multiple roles and settings required of an OB/Gyn, such as office pacing, results management, management of mid-levels, and efficient documentation. Attempting to transition to these roles and tasks while also teaching can be overwhelming. In addition, while it is hard to develop the respect and trust of one's peers when in a new setting, it can be much harder when you are a teacher and your learners are close to you in age, leading to a potential higher risk of imposter syndrome in young attendings working in academic settings.

If you decide to choose an academic career, how do you set yourself up for success? To succeed in academics, one first needs to assess their values. Do you want to primarily be a researcher or clinician? Do you love working with residents but have trouble relating to medical students? Do you thrive in leadership roles or do they add undue stress? Before you accept an academic position, you need to think through these questions and ensure that the job being offered provides the ideal balance of education, research, leadership and clinical work; this will vary greatly by individual. Once you accept your "ideal" job with the perfect ratio of these roles, live in it for several years. No job is perfect, and you will eventually find you need to titrate these ratios to better fit your interests or life stage.

Those who succeed in academics are always reassessing the best balance between patient safety, learner autonomy, and self-development. It might be safe for patients to always have a senior attending physician perform their operation, but then we will inadequately develop the hands-on surgical skills of our next generation of surgeons. A resident might want to do a hysterectomy themselves from start to finish, but a patient who has four prior cesarean sections might not be the best patient for them to have as their first solo hysterectomy. The attending physician might want to do a vaginal delivery themselves because it is a patient whom they have delivered two times before, but a straightforward multiparous delivery is likely to be an ideal learning case for a student or lower-level resident. The balance between needs constantly shifts, and those who are successful in academic medicine are able to continually reassess the balance.

In summary, it is important to weigh the benefits and downsides of academic medicine before choosing this path. If teaching excites and invigorates you, this may be the path for you. If you think you would want to start practice in a place where you have more independence and autonomy, then perhaps a non-academic position is a better fit. It is important to realize that even if you choose to start on a non-academic path, you can always choose to change to academics later in your career when you are more established, financially and as a clinician. Then, once you choose academics, consider which ratio of roles would best allow you to thrive. Lastly, recognize that the job description you start with will need to change and will likely go through many iterations as your career progresses and your personal needs and interests change.

Chapter 19
Laborist and OB-GYN Hospitalist Positions

Michelle Salvatore

Introduction

The energy of the labor floor is often one of the most compelling parts of the field of OB-GYN. Choosing to focus your career on becoming an OB Laborist or OB Hospitalist is an exciting career path. This unique area provides the opportunity for the Obstetricians to practice obstetrics at a higher level and collaborate to achieve the best patient care.

The Concept of an OB Laborist/OB-GYN Hospitalist

Our colleagues in Internal Medicine first codified the concept of a hospitalist. Hospitalist physicians focus their practice on the inpatient setting. Their focus includes patient care, inpatient teaching, and participation on hospital committees. The scope of practice encompasses admissions and consults in the emergency department, floor consults, escalation to critical care, coordination of care, and establishment of post-hospitalization care to name a few. From this foundation came the concept of the Obstetric and Gynecologic Hospitalist.

A hospital-only practice model for OBGYN was developed in the early 2000s. As an OBGYN Hospitalist, the primary role is to care for obstetric patients in the hospital and manage obstetric emergencies. Typically, this is off-set with little to no outpatient and elective GYN surgery responsibilities, though many OBGYN Hospitalists provide emergency GYN consultation and GYN surgical care.

There are various practice models utilizing OBGYN Hospitalist providers. In some, the OBGYN Hospitalist may replace having other OBGYNs in the hospital

M. Salvatore (✉)
Virtua Health, Marlton, NJ, USA

A. Malik et al. (eds.), *An Obstetrician/Gynecologist's Path*,
https://doi.org/10.1007/978-3-031-87098-9_19

and completely manage all inpatients regardless of where they get their prenatal care. In other models, the OBGYN Hospitalist assists and compliments the traditional full-scope OBGYN providers. Each model has unique roles and responsibilities for the OBGYN Hospitalist, which is often dependent on the specific health system. Some settings may have more focus on OB and less on GYN, while others may be a pure 50/50 mix.

OBGYN Hospitalist Roles and Responsibilities

Let's take a closer look at the roles and responsibilities of an OB-GYN Hospitalist. Common OB responsibilities include the triage of obstetric patients presenting to the hospital, care for unassigned patients, admission of patients for labor or induction or cesarean section, antepartum admissions, and management of labor. The OB-GYN Hospitalist provides assistance with operative vaginal deliveries, shoulder dystocia cases, and complex cesarean section cases, such as accreta spectrum and multiple gestation.

The management of obstetric emergencies is a key role of the OB-GYN Hospitalist. Some examples of these are precipitous deliveries, postpartum hemorrhage, expedited management of acute hypertension, magnesium toxicity, respiratory compromise, and any rapid response attention needed by obstetric patients in the hospital. For this reason, it is imperative that the OB-GYN Hospitalist be experienced in these acute situations and comfortable with hospital protocols and safety bundles to safely lead the team and care for the obstetric emergency. The OB-GYN Hospitalist acts as the glue of the Labor and Delivery unit by being versed in effective resource use and must have a focus on quality metrics like primary cesarean section and episiotomy rates. They maintain a culture of communication, quality, and safety by bridging providers and nursing. The OB-GYN Hospitalist often participates in maternal child health interdisciplinary committees to improve care delivery and management of obstetric emergencies.

Teaching Focus

Qualifications

Excellent candidates for OB-GYN Hospitalist are Board Certified and can demonstrate experience with management of acute and emergent obstetric care. Most programs prefer a minimum of 3–5 years of prior full scope OB-GYN experience. There are some fellowships available that are focused on training to be an OBGYN Hospitalist, which are especially useful for newer physicians. Each hospital may have specifications related to position requirements.

Fellowships

As noted, there are a few available fellowships for OBGYN Hospitalist. Most are 2-year programs with advanced education in hospital-based obstetrics and gynecology focused on patient safety. These programs have a blend of clinical, surgical, and healthcare systems training. Some provide experience in both academic and community-based hospital settings. The fellowships are designed for physicians specifically interested in gaining skills in hospital obstetric medicine. The programs also focus on leadership growth.

Fellowship responsibilities often include providing patient care, teaching clinical activities, and demonstrating professional competency. Programs offer experience in managing critical care obstetrics as well as management of emergency gynecologic procedures. The fellowships offer exposure to low-risk and complex high-risk pregnancies and the management of medical, obstetrical, and surgical complications affecting these patients. There is a focus on the multidisciplinary approach to obstetric patient care across antepartum, intrapartum, and postpartum periods. Fellows improve their procedural skills in areas such as complex laceration repair, operative vaginal delivery, and peripartum hysterectomy.

Fellowship is not required for all OB-GYN Hospitalist positions. Again, the skilled and experienced OB-GYN with a focus in this area is well suited for these clinical roles. Newer graduates from OB-GYN residency can greatly benefit from this type of focused critical care obstetric training fellowship.

OB-GYN Hospitalist Program Benefits

There are obvious benefits for the health system, the patients, and the providers when utilizing OB-GYN Hospitalist programs. The foremost benefits are quality and safety. OBGYN Hospitalists provide consistent physician coverage and standardization of care. Additionally, hospitalists typically work in shifts, instead of long 24–36 hours of continuous call-time, and reduced fatigue has been shown to lead to improved outcomes. The reduction in fatigue also is associated with less burn-out. The schedule of an OB-GYN Hospitalist is much like an Emergency Department Physician with predictable hours, assigned shifts, and fewer unanticipated clinical responsibilities. This practice model contributes to lifestyle satisfaction and wellness that many OBGYN physicians seek. In addition, many OB-GYN Hospitalist physicians use non-shift time to develop and participate in leadership activities in the health system. The OB-GYN Hospitalist has become a popular model of care as OB-GYN physicians look to balance work, career development, and personal life. The collaborative model lends benefits to the OBGYN Hospitalist and to our full-scope OBGYN colleagues in traditional practice. Future outcomes research, both quantitative and qualitative, should help to solidify the effectiveness of such OBGYN Hospitalist programs.

Society of OB/GYN Hospitalists

The Society of OB/GYN Hospitalists was formed in 2011 and is a large network of OB/GYN Hospitalist providers. Members are inclusive of physicians, midwives, nurses, and other healthcare professionals. For more information on the Society of OB/GYN Hospitalists, please visit https://societyofobgynhospitalists.org/.

Bibliography

1. American College of Obstetricians and Gynecologists' Committee on Patient Safety and Quality Improvement; American College of Obstetricians and Gynecologists' Committee on Obstetric Practice. ACOG Committee Opinion No. 657: the obstetric and gynecologic hospitalist. Obstet Gynecol. 2016;127(2):e81-5.
2. https://societyofobgynhospitalists.org/

Chapter 20
Joining Private Practice

Cosette Gabriel

So you've decided on a career in private practice… congratulations! You might be attracted to private practice for the flexibility, or perhaps even the prospect of becoming partner/owner. The endeavor can seem daunting at first and there are certainly important aspects to consider. Private practice in obstetrics and gynecology has continually evolved over the last several years. There has been a growing movement toward employment over private practice, largely due to increased cost of professional liability coverage, increased burnout in the field, and employee benefits such as health insurance and retirement matching. Despite these considerations, a job in private practice can be truly rewarding. This chapter offers important points to consider when joining a private practice.

I began my job search at the end of my third year of residency. My husband and I are both in medicine and we had decided not to pursue any fellowship opportunities. This left us with the decision to stay in academic medicine, such as a hospital-based practice, or join private practice. With hospital-based practices, you are typically an employee of a hospital or health system, but these options can vary greatly. These positions can involve research and teaching, involve typical weekday shifts and call opportunities, and can sometimes offer additional funds for call. Often, these positions can provide more stability and take away some of the stress about the financial operations of a practice. Although the growing landscape of medicine has shifted toward hospital-based practice, we were largely motivated to join private practice due to the flexibility and the prospect of "being your own boss."

In private practice and OB/GYN especially, a large number of practices are now owned by private equity. Private equity allows you to work for a company that is focused on the financial return of the medical practice. This can be very appealing to applicants, and these positions are often able to offer higher starting salaries and

C. Gabriel (✉)
Contemporary Women's Care, Orlando, FL, USA

UCF Lake Nona Hospital, Orlando, FL, USA

A. Malik et al. (eds.), *An Obstetrician/Gynecologist's Path*,
https://doi.org/10.1007/978-3-031-87098-9_20

signing bonuses. These positions can be financially rewarding and offer some flexibility. Some of these positions may even offer partnership opportunities; however, they often do not offer true ownership tracks and the flexibility that comes with it. Asking about partnership and ownership opportunities up front can help you to shape your long-term goals and understand what your future at a particular practice might look like.

Before I started interviewing, I thought about my ideal work week. While clinic time in residency is typically minimal compared to hospital-based care, I knew that joining private practice would be the complete opposite. While interviewing, I was vocal to recruiters and practices that I eventually desired about one day per week on Labor and Delivery, one day for surgery, and the remainder of my work week in clinic seeing patients. I understood that this type of schedule would take time to build as I built my brand and patient base, but I looked for a group that would be supportive of this schedule.

Knowing that most of my time would be spent in clinic, I sought to understand how clinic is run and what the practice does to ensure efficiency. Important considerations include appointment length for new versus established patients, how procedures are incorporated into the schedule, and confirmation of pregnancy visits. I was interested in the quality of equipment at the office, including a dedicated ultrasound and capability to perform in-office procedures. Over the course of interviewing, it became important to me that the practice provide support staff assigned specifically to my schedule to ensure appropriate appointment times and time between complex and straightforward visits. I also asked about expectations for delivering results to patients and if support staff helped with this responsibility.

It is important to ask how the clinic operates on your call day. In my current practice, we take home calls and providers are only scheduled prenatal visits and preventive exams on call days so that they can easily be rescheduled or seen by another provider that same day. I made sure to understand how after-hour calls and questions get delivered to the on-call provider, namely, do these calls go directly to the on-call provider or are they triaged by an answering service? I also made sure to inquire about who fields patients calls and questions during the workday.

With regard to call responsibilities, most private practices take home call. The exception to this is if you join a large volume private practice, which may require in-house call. Home call allows the physician to remain in the clinic during the workday and continues to be probably the most challenging aspect for me to juggle as a new attending. Actively managing patients to deliver at convenient times during the workday is an art that I continue to learn from my partners. It is also important to know who sees triage patients while taking home call—is there an OB Hospitalist that your practice has an agreement with, or a certified nurse midwife/nurse practitioner/physician assistant? These ancillary staff can help minimize interruptions to patient care during your call days.

The moment I signed my contract, I breathed a sigh of relief. I began to get excited about starting my new job and thought about what kind of attending I wanted to be. I realized very quickly upon starting that there was a large part of my job that is customer service and marketing. I had to learn who the referring primary care physicians in the area are, as well as the subspecialists who I would be referring my patients to. One of the ways to familiarize yourself with the community is to work with your Physician Relations Director to meet other physicians in the community. In my case, this is an individual employed by the hospital whose purpose is to help you build and maintain relationships with other physicians within the hospital system, as well as serve as the point person for any concerns. Though the exact title and function of this person can vary among hospital systems, there is usually an individual who the practice may rely on to serve this function and would be an important person to seek out. Outside of this, I make it a point to introduce myself to other physicians in the Doctor's Lounge at the hospital. My practice also sent out email blasts to our referring physicians introducing me as the newest member of the team and used social media to introduce me to patients.

Patients read reviews and want to see a provider that they feel comfortable with, trust with their care, and who will deliver results in a timely fashion. In our field, patients especially want a clean office with appropriate privacy and staff that are polite and professional. Going the extra mile to build trust and rapport with your patients will only attract more patients. I make it a point to call my patients in the postoperative period to check on them and see how they are doing. I also call patients with sensitive results instead of sending a message on the patient portal or having a support staff member deliver these. The few additional minutes spent communicating with patients directly has made the biggest impact on their trust in me. These are all things that will grow your practice and establish your reputation in the community.

Transitioning away from residency where you often feel like a "resident" of the hospital toward private practice where you spend the majority of time in the office can feel like a huge shift. Emphasis on clinical duties, time management, and building your brand of medicine can be very different from residency in academic or even community settings. Ultimately, private practice can provide an opportunity to practice ob/gyn independently and undertake the business of medicine, while enjoying flexibility of schedule and financial benefits of partnership/ownership.

Part III
After Starting Your First Job

Chapter 21
Dealing with Your Clinic

Simone Sweeney

Congratulations. You have completed residency and possibly fellowship and have successfully secured employment. Whether you are in an academic or private setting, you will more likely than not spend a portion of your time seeing patients in the outpatient clinic. The ambulatory setting is where you will encounter the majority of your patients, some of which will become long-term established patients. This chapter is an overview of managing the outpatient office, as well as a few tips and tricks for specific situations.

When you are vetting an institution, you should ask relevant questions regarding the clinic. What are the working hours? Are there opportunities for early or late hours? How many clinic sessions are you expected to complete on a weekly basis? How many patients are you expected to see on a daily basis? Are you able to adjust your template to accommodate more complex patients? Make sure you are comfortable with the answer to these questions prior to accepting the position.

Once you officially start your position, you will be assigned an office location and introduced to the staff. Now, understanding the ambulatory dynamic is important and usually pretty standard regardless if the practice is established or brand new. There is an office manager who runs the clinic. This person is responsible for budget, equipment, medications, vaccinations, personnel, schedules, etc. The office assistant manages the patient scheduling and clerical duties for the office. The medical assistants will arrange your patient rooms, room the patients, and directly assist with your patient examinations. As the provider, you'll need to establish a great relationship with all of these people to ensure that your office runs smoothly. Be specific about your needs and check in when you feel there is room for improvement.

S. Sweeney (✉)
Department of Obstetrics and Gynecology, Cooper Medical School of Rowan University and Cooper University Health Care, Camden, NJ, USA

A. Malik et al. (eds.), *An Obstetrician/Gynecologist's Path*,
https://doi.org/10.1007/978-3-031-87098-9_21

After meeting the staff, tour the office and familiarize yourself with the layout. Where are the providers' offices? Where do the medical assistants sit? Find the bathrooms and the lunchroom. Explore the patient rooms BEFORE you see a patient in them. How do you raise and lower the beds? Where's the light source? Where are the speculums and lubricant located? How do you notify your MA that you need a chaperone?

Next, shadowing! Following an established provider (if possible) for a few days can be extremely insightful. You'll learn the flow of the office, see how certain diagnoses or visit types are billed and freshen up on your medical decision-making. This is also an opportunity for you to ask questions! That is, how do I refer for colonoscopy? What about lactation?

If you are working at an institution other than where you completed residency, you will be required to do training on your hospital's EMR during onboarding. Although this training is helpful, it will not be enough for you to become proficient. During your first few weeks, you will need to spend extra time familiarizing yourself with the EMR, saving frequent diagnoses, and creating order sets, smart phrases, and note templates. This will help you to be more efficient when you begin seeing a full patient panel. Don't be afraid to ask for an abbreviated schedule. During this period of transition, you should ask to see less patients while you adjust to the EMR and office flow, until you can increase your speed and efficiency.

Prep your charts! When you are a new provider, all patients will be new to you, even if they are established within the clinic. So you should review all relevant medical history, medications, and surgeries before meeting the patient. Writing down these details, whether using a sticky note feature or in the pre-charting context, will remove the need for you to remember specifics. You can also pend orders, for example, prenatal labs for a new pregnancy or a screening mammogram for a routine well woman exam. This allows for a better patient interaction and efficiency.

You should strive to complete your documentation the same day. If you prepped your charts as recommended, you should have some basic information already completed in your patient note. Complete the HPI during the patient encounter when possible. This will allow you to use the patient's words, and you will not have to recall specifics since they are already written down. Given the modern medical system, many patients expect that you will interface with the computer screen during the visit. Order any labs, imaging, or medication before starting the physical exam when possible. Ask the patient if they need a refill of medications or if they would accept appropriate imaging based on their complaint before you transition to the hands on portion of the visit. After you complete the patient interaction, document the physical exam portion so you can mention any abnormal findings. If there is not enough time to complete the note before your next patient encounters, insert your diagnoses and place key words in your plan. This will allow you to remember the treatment plan you discussed when you return to complete the note.

After a few weeks have gone by and you are seeing patients regularly, this means you are ordering labs and imaging that will need to be reviewed. These results will also need to be relayed to the patient in a timely fashion. Discuss whether your medical assistant or nurse will assist with results. If you are calling patients to review results, make sure to document these encounters. If you are unable to reach patients with a critical result, make sure to send a certified result (typically done via a letter sent via certified mail) and document this.

Similar to labs and imaging, most EMRs now allow patients to send provider messages. You'll need to incorporate time into your schedule to address these. Most of the messages you will be able to address quickly; however, others may require more time. Consider responding to all your messages at the beginning of the day or at the end of each session; however, you may want to avoid answering them mid-session, as this can interrupt workflow and disrupt patient care. Setting aside time for responses to patients can help prevent build up, which can be overwhelming for providers. Some institutions will have a fielding process where messages are reviewed and addressed by nurses first, then sent to the provider if necessary. In this case, make sure your nurse is aware of your preferences. Review how you would respond to commonly asked questions and which concerns should be brought to you. Empower your nurse to ask questions and include them in responses to patients. They will learn from you and ultimately rely on you less.

Now, let's discuss tips for specific clinic scenarios.

Absences

There should be a plan in place to deal with your absence, whether it is scheduled vacation or a last-minute emergency. Communication is key in this scenario. Make sure your office manager is aware in advance of any scheduled time away from the office. This allows for appropriate scheduling and provider coverage if needed. Remember that it is still your responsibility to manage your inbox! So if you do not plan on monitoring it while away or will have limited internet access, arrange for another provider to cover your inbox BEFORE you leave. In the case of an emergency, your office staff should be told as soon as possible. Your staff should contact the scheduled patients and reschedule them. In group practices, patients can be diverted to other providers' schedules if possible. If feasible, you can consider adding or lengthening another session to accommodate patients who had their appointments canceled.

Collaboration with Other Providers

You will work with other providers within and outside your specialty regularly in the outpatient setting. This is beneficial for several reasons. First, your colleagues can assist with diagnosis. Maybe your patient has a rash that you have not encountered before or they've failed a treatment plan and you are having difficulty creating a new one. Our colleagues have different experiences than we do and may be able to offer an alternative you haven't considered (or validate a decision you already made).

Co-management and clearances are other opportunities for collaboration. You will have patients in both the obstetric and gynecologic sector that have other comorbidities. Your colleagues in other specialties can manage the issues that are not quite in your scope of practice. This is also helpful when preoperative clearances or medication adjustments are needed for surgical procedures. Responding promptly and professionally to messages from colleagues is important for managing these interdepartmental relationships and can help ensure they are mutually beneficial. Showing respect and being communicative can often be rewarded with referrals. Providers will refer their patients to other providers that they have interacted with and can trust.

Dealing with the Difficult Patient

Patients can be termed "difficult" for several reasons. Maybe they have a complex medical history or a more aggressive temperament. Either way, there are a few tricks to navigating these interactions. First, *be pleasant*! A friendly smile and greeting sets the tone for a good visit and can help head off negative interactions. *Be familiar with the patient's history when possible*. This is where your chart prep can be extremely helpful. *Allow the patient to speak*. "Difficult" patients typically complain of not feeling heard or listened to. Allow them to express their concerns while actively listening. This is where adjusting your schedule for more complex patients can come in handy; it is easier to allow adequate time to listen when you know there aren't several patients waiting for you. *Address their concerns to the best of your ability*. Review the workup and potential treatment options. Verbalize to the patient your thought process, and why certain tests may be beneficial or not. *Last, be honest*. Can you help this patient? Do they need a sub-specialist or a different specialty altogether? Do not feel like you have to solve everything if it is out of your scope.

Same-Day Visits, Urgent and Emergent Care

There will be instances where patients will request a same-day appointment—time to use those triaging skills from residency. If you determine that this patient has an emergent need such as decreased fetal movement or vaginal bleeding in pregnancy, make sure to direct them to the hospital for emergent evaluation. If a patient is experiencing acute symptoms such as vaginal discharge or dysuria, you can attempt to accommodate these patients as your schedule allows.

Self-collection is also an option if that is offered by your specific clinic. If unable to accommodate a patient in this manner, you can consider directing your patient to an urgent care where the acute symptom can be addressed prior to being evaluated by you.

Insurance Companies: Prior Authorizations and Peer to Peers

Some medications and imaging studies will require prior authorizations. These can be filed automatically at time of prescribing or may need to be filed manually. The majority of the time the insurance company just requires additional information before approving the request. Make sure to support your decision-making in your documentation since they will request supporting progress notes as needed; this can also allow ancillary staff to help complete prior authorizations on your behalf. Peer to peer conversations are your chance to verbally defend your decision-making. These are easy to schedule and usually only take a few minutes. As long as you are able to defend your order when speaking with your peer, the majority of these decisions will be in your favor.

Case Collection

In the first few years of practice, most Ob-Gyns are preparing for board certification. There is an office practice portion of the exam which you should consider when treating your patients.

You should always practice evidence-based medicine; however, make sure that your actions will also be defendable when you sit for oral boards.

Overall, the outpatient clinic is an adventure filled with fulfilling patient interactions and fun working relationships. Embrace the journey and you'll thrive.

Best of luck!

Chapter 22
Building a Program

Robert L. Hunter

Pursuing a career in obstetrics and gynecology can seem very straightforward. You can choose to be a generalist, or you can obtain a fellowship in one of the many subspecialties of obstetrics and gynecology. The scope of practice within these disciplines of obstetrics and gynecology is well established. What is often less apparent is that you have the ability to carve out a niche for yourself within your chosen area of practice and create a program. For instance, if you have a particular interest in vaginitis, you may want to establish a vaginitis center of excellence. Alternatively, you may find that the needs of your community are not being met and adding a service or specialty program is beneficial for the health and well-being of your local patient population. You may therefore want to develop a Placenta Accreta Spectrum program or implement an Obstetrical Emergency Department to service the patients in your region or health care system [1]. Regardless of the impetus to modify your scope of practice, understanding the process of building a niche program is necessary to affect change in a positive manner and meet your goals. The purpose of this chapter is to provide some guidance on how to successfully develop such a specialty program.

Developing a successful program requires several key steps. First, you must identify exactly what you are hoping to achieve, and secondly, why you have this objective. Once you can answer these two questions, you have the framework to define your mission and create a mission statement. While often difficult to craft,

R. L. Hunter (✉)
Department of Obstetrics and Gynecology at the Florida International University, Herbert Wertheim College of Medicine (FIU-HWCOM), Miami, FL, USA

Department of Obstetrics and Gynecology, Memorial Healthcare System, Hollywood, FL, USA

Acute Hospital Medicine, OB/GYN Hospitalist, TeamHealth, Knoxville, TN, USA

A. Malik et al. (eds.), *An Obstetrician/Gynecologist's Path*,
https://doi.org/10.1007/978-3-031-87098-9_22

developing a mission statement will help describe your purpose and keep you focused as you work to achieve your goal [4]. Since a new endeavor can be extremely challenging, your mission statement must center your process on the path to your endpoint and articulate a clear message regarding the reason for your existence. For example, Apple's mission statement is "to bring the best user experience to customers through innovative hardware, software, and services [6]." Apple's mission statement guides all of their product development and has informed their approach to create the best user experience for their customers. This mission-centered approach will also help you as you work to achieve buy-in to your program from key stakeholders. New initiatives are not built in isolation, as they require support from a wide array of personnel and service lines. A captivating and purposeful mission statement will facilitate securing support from others to help advance your program.

The next step in building a successful program is formulating the costs associated with this initiative. The costs should be defined by several factors:

- What is your budget?
- What are the upfront and ongoing equipment and material costs?
- What resources are needed in terms of personnel?
- How much will these employees cost per year in salary and benefits?
- What additional resources are required, such as marketing and advertising?
- What will the program cost per year beyond the start-up costs?
- What will the program be able to generate in terms of revenue?
- Will the program be able to achieve profitability, and if so, when?

Once the costs are defined, then you need to articulate the anticipated benefits of your program. Understanding these benefits will guide you as you gain support for this endeavor. Again, programs do not exist in isolation; they require the support of key personnel, such as hospital administration, community leaders, other service line professionals, and investors, to name a few. Finding synergy between the defined benefits of your program and the needs and motivations of these stakeholders will help you cultivate the necessary support to move your initiative forward [3].

While you may be excited about your new proposition, other colleagues around you might have a negative perspective and view the addition as an unwelcome change or a burden to their already busy professional lives. Being a leader of change requires patience and perseverance to take the time to obtain acceptance to an innovative idea or concept. Therefore, you need to project a clear message and demonstrate the benefits to the affected parties. Gaining support requires a great deal of organization and education to whom you are appealing for assistance. Remember to remain patient; answer all questions with grace, gratitude, and understanding; be open to suggestions; and be prepared to make compromises along the way.

Oftentimes, the vision and the end result are more important than the implementation details. Incorporating the ideas and suggestions of other individuals allows them to gain ownership in the program, which can result in strong allies and invested team members. Additionally, they may be open to executing a new program in stages, rather than all at once. This gradual approach makes the changes more palatable to those people most affected by the program. A systematic roll-out allows time for the benefits of the program to become apparent to the team and allows for course corrections in each stage, especially when faced with unintended consequences that inevitably arise.

One example is the creation of an Obstetrical Emergency Department staffed by physicians in a well-established community hospital, which has an existing Labor and Delivery Triage Unit run by a veteran nursing staff [2]. Building a new program, such as this Obstetrical Emergency Department, requires all of the efforts and ideas outlined in the above paragraphs. The first step is to define the what and the why. The "what" is the establishment of an Obstetrical Emergency Department (OB ED). The "why" is to improve upon the quality of care provided to pregnant patients with acute conditions, when they arrive at the hospital. Patient safety and quality of care should be at the heart of your messaging to hospital administration, the community physicians, nursing leadership, and the community. Gaining support for your initiative from hospital administration is often the first key to obtaining broader downstream acceptance. An OB ED program requires support from such departments as the main Emergency Department, blood bank, laboratory, imaging, and other critical service lines. Their input and participation is integral to the success of the unit, and these departments and their personnel have experience with emergency care, which is vital to the logistical planning necessary to building a successful OB ED.

Next, calculating the costs associated with the establishment of an OB ED is crucial. A clear understanding of the anticipated volume will help to determine the level of around-the-clock staffing with nursing and medical professionals you need to provide safe and timely care. Understanding the clinical volume and payer mix will help you estimate the expected professional and facility reimbursements, which will be collected to offset the cost of staffing. Understanding the rules and regulations associated with the establishment of an Emergency Department is also integral to ensure proper compliance, operation, and avoidance of fines or violations.

Anticipating challenges to your program implementation is equally vital. You must think about who is most adversely affected by your program, and then work to alleviate their concerns and educate them on the expected benefits. In the OB ED example, the community physicians and the nursing staff would be most expected to express resistance, because they are the key drivers of the traditional Triage Unit and may perceive this change as an indictment of the care they were providing. Positive messaging is essential to alleviating these concerns. Also, gradual execution may allow the nursing staff and community physicians to adjust to the change and provide input along the way. Slow implementation can further allow them to see the benefits first hand. For nursing, they might benefit from having a physician readily available to deal with an emergency, such as a patient presenting with a bleeding previa or an abruption. The community physicians, who may enjoy getting less calls while at home, may also appreciate the security of having a board-certified obstetrician performing a medical screening exam on their patients in person in an acute setting.

Other programs may present additional challenges. Another example is the establishment of a Placenta Accreta Spectrum program [5]. This high-risk program may take significant effort to convince the interested parties that the community benefits of the program are worth the medical and legal risks. Implementing a high-risk program such as a Placenta Accreta Spectrum program also presents a learning curve. Outcomes improve with experience on the part of the participating team members (Obstetricians, Trauma or Gynecologic Oncology specialists, Maternal Fetal Medicine specialists, Anesthesia, OR nursing, Blood Bank, etc.), yet while the team is gaining experience, poor patient outcomes could occur. The solution is to emphasize the long-term positive value of developing a challenging program that can overcome a gap in care for patients in the community with abnormal placentation. However, this type of program not only benefits the community members but also serves as a resource for other obstetricians in the region, who may not be equipped to handle these cases in their institutions. A Placenta Accreta Program can raise the level of care in the region and add prestige to the sponsoring institution.

Another factor to consider when deciding to build a program is the effort you need to gain the mandatory clinical expertise to run a program and market yourself as an expert. As a health professional, you have to commit to patient safety and quality, which may demand additional education such as going to conferences or working under another expert. For example, if you would like to start a vaginitis center, you have to acquire the expertise necessary to provide a level of care that other gynecologists are unable to provide. In addition, building a successful program requires word of mouth support from patients and referrals from other providers. Delivering quality and expertise should be at the heart of this endeavor.

The practice of medicine is a life-long commitment to education and growth. As your practice evolves, you have the opportunity to explore areas of interest that tap into your expertise and the needs of the patients you serve. Therefore, recognizing how to build a program that meets your practice goals is critical. While the expertise necessary to provide quality care is vital to the success of your new program, understanding how to introduce change, message succinctly, work with others, and embrace their input is equally important. This chapter serves to offer a framework on how to build a successful program to achieve personal and professional satisfaction and serve the needs of your community.

References

1. Tussey C, Olson C. Creating a multidisciplinary placenta accreta program. Nurs Womens Health. 2018;22(5):372–86.
2. Hunter R. Change management: enhancing OB/GYN care in a Florida health system, case study. 2022. TeamHealth.com.
3. Zeh HJ III. Building a successful clinical program in the academic medical center. In: Surgical mentorship and leadership: building for success in academic surgery. Cham: Springer; 2018. p. 181–8.
4. Desmidt S, Prinzie AA. The organization's mission statement: give up hope or resuscitate? A search for evidence-based recommendations. Adv Health Care Manag. 2011;10:25–41. https://doi.org/10.1108/s1474-8231(2011)000001008.

5. ACOG Clinical Consensus. Placenta accreta spectrum, Number 7. December 2018, Reaffirmed 2021.
6. Pereira D. Apple mission and vision statement. The Business Model Analyst. 7 April 2023. https://businessmodelanalyst.com/apple-mission-and-vision-statement/.

Chapter 23
Navigating EMRs

Rori Dajao

Navigating EMRs

The term Electronic Medical Record (EMRs) is interchangeable with Electronic Health Record (EHRs). These are distinct from a Personal Health Record, where the patient is the primary custodian/controller of the information within it. The Centers for Medicare and Medicaid Services (CMS) defines "Electronic Health Records" as (emphasis mine):

> *...an electronic version of a patient's medical history, that is* ***maintained by the provider over time****, and may include all of the key administrative clinical data relevant to that person's care under a particular provider, including demographics, progress notes, problems, medications, vital signs, past medical history, immunizations, laboratory data and radiology reports. The EHR automates access to information and* ***has the potential to streamline the clinician's workflow****. The EHR also has the ability to support other care-related activities directly or indirectly through various interfaces, including evidence-based decision support, quality management, and outcomes reporting.*
>
> *EHRs are the next step in the continued progress of healthcare that* ***can strengthen the relationship between patients and clinicians.*** *The data, and the timeliness and availability of it, will enable providers to make better decisions and provide better care.*[1]

This definition is a great description of the multiple layers of possibility that a properly maintained EHR has for you, the patient, and the rest of the care team, and I will use it to structure this discussion.

[1] https://www.cms.gov/priorities/key-initiatives/e-health/records

R. Dajao (✉)
Department of Obstetrics and Gynecology, Cooper Medical School of Rowan University and Cooper University Health Care, Camden, NJ, USA

A. Malik et al. (eds.), *An Obstetrician/Gynecologist's Path*,
https://doi.org/10.1007/978-3-031-87098-9_23

"EMRs Are Maintained by the Provider Over Time…"

A patient's EMR is a true "garbage in, garbage out" system. It is purely and totally dependent on the quality of information that is placed within it. For EMRs, "quality" of information refers to both its accuracy and its actual location within the record. To illustrate this, a generational metaphor is helpful. I cannot remember where I heard this metaphor, but it truly crystallizes this notion of information storage for me. Being born in the late 1970s, I happen to span these two generations and am comfortable moving between both modes of thought. Older generations see themselves as "librarians" for their digital information, meaning that they think of information as being stored in specific places under a discrete file structure that they created and of which they are aware. Imagine a traditional library with shelves of physical media. There is a section for fiction, nonfiction, etc. Each book, DVD, magazine has a specific place in the library. As librarians, we know exactly where in the library each piece of information should be placed and therefore we know exactly where we need to go to obtain a piece of information. As a new attending, you had been likely brought up in the new generation of the "Search Bar." In this world, you are not the librarian. You are the person coming to purely access information, and you present a request for that information to the librarian who simply gives it to you. The library itself is a black box that you cannot see into. In their current state (as of December 2023), EMRs are structured in the "old" way of digital organization. So you need to know where things go. By placing information in its proper place, the most amount of people will have access to it. This is because the EMR itself does not yet know where to place the information. Many EMRs can find all the information you ask for, but if it is not placed in the right location, it might not be found, or worse, it could be reported wrongly. As we move into the newest generation of information technology, i.e., of artificial intelligence (AI), your EMR may be able to perform the active organization of information on its own, but we aren't there yet. So think of yourself as the actual librarian of your patient's EMR.

Finally, from a higher level perspective, if the library of each patient is well organized, it unlocks the advanced levels of functionality of your EMR. Large sets of data are easier to harvest when individual charts are well organized and standardized. This will enable your practice to create useful Best Practice Alerts and get quality improvement data that can be used to affect patient outcomes. For example, data collection can be automated if the initial data is input correctly, allowing your team to focus on root cause parts of a workflow that you are trying to improve sooner than if you had to review the same number of charts manually. Then once you have made your intervention to process, compliance with the process is easier to track with the automated review that you have already created.

"An EMR Has the Potential to Streamline the Clinician's Workflow…"

I was lucky enough to train at and now work for a system where the EMR was the same both in the inpatient and outpatient settings. This means that my notes from my clinic are visible to me when I am managing the patient when they are admitted to the hospital. If you are still considering several job offers, this kind of arrangement should be given a lot of weight on the "pro" side of the equation. The efficiency that this arrangement allows results in an enormous quality of life benefit for you as a provider, and it just makes it easier to take care of the patient. To use our generational metaphor, it is the same library for both inpatients and outpatients as opposed to two separate libraries.

You will continue to use an EMR every day for the rest of your career, so efficiency is key. During your residency training, it is likely that your use of the EMR had inefficiencies baked into your workflow based on your level of training. Additionally, it is likely that outpatient medicine played only a small role in your weekly schedule. However, as a generalist OB/Gyn attending, your schedule will suddenly be very (very) outpatient heavy. You will go from seeing 30 patients a week to seeing 30 patients a day. This can lead to burnout, inducing a sense of disillusionment. On the other hand, in an outpatient-heavy world, timelines for care now stretch to weeks to months instead of minutes to hours as they are in an inpatient setting. Because of this time dilation, you may feel like you have more time to document things. Technically you do, but since your patient volume is going to rise dramatically, the number of charts that you now must deal with is much greater. To address this load, I am firmly in the "Pre-Charting" camp.

A typical schedule for an 8-hour day is 30 patients scheduled every 15 minutes with a 1-hour break for lunch. Your no-show rate as an attending will be much lower than it was as a resident, so you can bank on seeing at least 95% of your schedule. That is a lot of talking throughout the day, and at the end of it, patients can all blend together. So instead of spending my time outside of the office *finishing* documentation for a *past* appointment, I strive to *start* documentation for a *future* appointment. Most EMRs have a Pre-Charting feature, where you can start the note, and even pend orders. Scheduling comments in your schedule should give you an idea of why the patient is coming to see you. Using these in concert, you can write a note so that it is 80–90% done as you are walking into the room. Doing this also gets you to delve a bit into the patient's chart ahead of time to see things from the patient's history that can drive the discussion. This way while you are speaking with the patient, you can just fill in the blanks of your prewritten note, and then as you are walking out of the room, you can sign the note and close the chart. This way your brain is "turned off" to the patient until the results of testing come back to you—more on this later. Additionally, knowing things about the patient's history ahead of time instills confidence in the patient. It feels different to the patient when you know these things, as opposed as them seeing you learn about them in real time as you click through their chart. Most patient satisfaction surveys (which may be used to calculate incentive bonuses) have a question such as "Did the provider know information from your medical chart before the start of the visit?"

Annual visits and New Patient visits (problem or annual) should be seen as a time for the tidying-up of your library—make sure that all the "books of information" are on the correct shelves, and all facing the right way. Be obsessive and systematic about it. Make sure that all the surgeries, especially abdominal ones, are in the Past Surgical History area of the EMR. Make sure that "migraine with aura" is in the Past Medical History area of the EMR. Both of those pieces of information can be free-typed into your note, but then it is known only to you in that note at that singular point in time, and not to every OB/Gyn (or PCP, or Neurologist, or Colorectal Surgeon) who has access to the patient's chart. Fix any automated parts of the chart that output information to the patient: if your EMR has a patient portal that reminds patients when they should get a pap smear, make sure it is at the correct interval based on the patient's age and insurance coverage. Input information that limits the number of keystrokes that you need to perform for that information both now and into the future: "Married 5 years" must be continually updated, while "current partner since 2018" can be simply verbally verified once input. If this is done routinely, all your subsequent visits with the patient will get faster and faster.

Finally, to streamline your visits even more, use the "private" area in a patient's EMR to communicate with yourself in the future. Most EMRs have a feature that allows you to make a note of something nonmedically related that only you can see, and that is associated with the patient's chart. Use this to make a note of little personal things that you spoke with the patient about (a trip that they just took, a life milestone, a funny joke, etc.), or maybe any special things that you need to do during the pelvic exam (like use a long speculum) to make the next exam quicker and easier for you and the patient.

"EMRs Can Strengthen the Relationship Between Patients and Clinicians…"

So, if you are successful at pre-charting an entire 30-patient schedule and are then able to close all 30 charts as you are leaving the room, as mentioned earlier, your brain can be turned off to the patient and you can then spend your free time in the evening preparing for the next session instead of remembering what happened over those previous 8 hours. Eventually, one by one, all the tests and procedures that you ordered for the patients will start arriving in your EMR inbox. If your patient's EMR is like a library, treat your EMR inbox like a haystack. Don't let it get too big! The vast majority of your inbox will be filled with normal and negative results. If this haystack gets too big, the abnormal and positive needles will be much more difficult to find, and it will take you longer to react to them (which could be a malpractice suit in the making).

Hopefully, your EMR has a patient portal. If it does, promote its use early and often to your patients. Have your support staff do the same. If you set expectations early (such as when you meet the patient for the very first time) that the portal is the best and most efficient way to exchange information with you, it will make your life much easier. The alternative is phone calls to patients who can take up much more of your time and energy—remember that there may be 30 more patients to see tomorrow! So sell your portal to the patients, and then actively use it. Lab results are now instantly available to patients as the results come in. If your portal message about the result comes soon after or better yet before they see it, it will put the patient at ease and make them believe that you are on the ball. When they ask you a question through the portal, respond promptly to it. If these interactions are performed over the portal, several interactions can occur simultaneously. I tell patients that they will hear good and bad news from me via the portal. I will say that this is so that they can get their results as quick as possible and that they can move onto the next step (treatment, specialist referral, etc.) sooner. I'll then say that this is how I get my own information from my physicians, and they usually accept that. Once they start seeing how fast I get back to them, and how much detail I can put into my responses they are extremely satisfied.

Becoming facile with your EMR can also help strengthen your relationships with the support people in your office—this is your new Work Family—because as a generalist, attending your time ensconced in the OB Workroom is over. Now you will be in an office most days where you may be the only physician in the office, or in an office where your partner is also trying to see 30 (or more) patients in 8 hours. Responding to a vaginitis result over the portal, ordering the Flagyl for BV electronically over the portal will relieve your office staff of that burden, and then make them more available for more important tasks to keep the office running as smoothly as possible.

The EMR is ubiquitous in healthcare, and at the end of the day, required. You should consider navigating and using your EMR skills as important as knot tying. It's the same type of skill—something that you do countless times a day without thinking that has the potential to do real harm to a patient if not done appropriately. Being a good steward of your patient's information in as efficient a way as possible makes caring for them as safe as possible.

Chapter 24
Enhancing Patient Experience in Obstetrics and Gynecology

Stephen Trzeciak and Anthony Mazzarelli

What Is Patient Experience?

Patient experience encompasses all aspects of a patient's interactions with the healthcare system, including their care from doctors, nurses, and staff in hospitals, physician practices, other healthcare facilities, and health plans. It reflects the entire range of interactions that patients undergo in the healthcare system, encompassing quality of care, clinical outcomes, interpersonal relationships, and communications, including those that involve intense emotion. Patient experience is a vital and distinct dimension of healthcare quality and involves several components, such as timely appointments, easy access to information, and good communication with healthcare providers. Clinician compassion has always been considered a cornerstone of high-quality patient experience, but it is also an important factor in patient outcomes.

Unlike the historical concept of "patient satisfaction," which can be subjective and based solely on patient expectations, the current framework of patient experience focuses on the delivery of healthcare services and objectively measures the extent to which patients are engaged in their care, the ease of access to healthcare services, and the quality of the environment in which they receive their care. We begin by defining elements of patient experience within the OB/GYN context, and then explain its critical role in patient retention, patient adherence to prescribed treatment, and the overall effectiveness of the health system.

S. Trzeciak (✉) · A. Mazzarelli
Cooper Medical School of Rowan University and Cooper University Health Care, Camden, NJ, USA

A. Malik et al. (eds.), *An Obstetrician/Gynecologist's Path*,
https://doi.org/10.1007/978-3-031-87098-9_24

Patient Experience in OB/GYN

In the field of OB/GYN, patient experience holds unique considerations, given the deeply personal and often sensitive nature of the care involved. OB/GYN practitioners support patients through some of the most significant moments over the course of their lives, e.g., childbirth and menopause, making compassionate, patient-centered care crucial. The ability of practitioners to build trust and establish strong, empathetic relationships is fundamental, as patients must feel comfortable discussing personal, perhaps intimate, matters of their health. Compassionate care can alleviate patient anxieties associated with reproductive health concerns, pregnancy, and any procedures that may be necessary.

Additionally, continuity of care is especially important in OB/GYN. Patients may benefit greatly from having a consistent caregiver or team throughout their reproductive years, enhancing the understanding and management of their long-term health needs. Moreover, the physical environment of OB/GYN clinics and hospitals plays a significant role. Spaces that ensure privacy and dignity during examinations and treatments contribute positively to the patient experience. Overall, enhancing patient experience in OB/GYN not only can improve patient outcomes but also fosters a supportive and empowering environment for patients at all stages of life.

Enhancing patient experience in OB/GYN also involves addressing the diverse needs of women across different life stages and cultural backgrounds. This requires practitioners to be culturally competent and sensitive to the varied beliefs, values, and practices related to reproductive health, childbirth, and gynecological care. Personalizing care to reflect a patient's cultural and individual preferences can significantly improve their engagement with the healthcare process. Patient education is another critical element in OB/GYN care, where informed patients are better equipped to make decisions about their reproductive health and treatment options. Providing accessible, understandable information about conditions, procedures, and preventive practices empowers women, leading to improved health outcomes and enhanced trust in the healthcare provider.

The Science Behind Compassionate Care

Compassion is defined as an emotional response to another person's pain, suffering, or struggle involving an authentic desire to help. It is distinct from a closely related term, "empathy." Empathy is the detecting, feeling, and understanding component. Compassion goes beyond empathy because it involves taking responsive action to alleviate another person's pain, suffering, or struggle, to whatever extent may be possible. Of course, empathy is essential to compassion, because if we do not detect or understand others' pain, we will miss every opportunity to respond to them with compassion. You can think of it like this: empathy + action = compassion.

The distinction is not just a matter of semantics. There are robust neuroscience data supporting this distinction in terms. Research using functional magnetic resonance imaging (MRI) has shown that when we bear witness to pain and suffering (empathy), it activates what neuroscience researchers consider a "pain center" of the brain. You also know this experientially because it is part of the reason why it is so uncomfortable to watch people suffer. Accordingly, there are neuroscience data behind the saying "I feel your pain." In contrast, when our mind is focused on taking action to help alleviate another person's pain or suffering, a distinctly different neural structure is activated on functional MRI scans. It is what neuroscience researchers consider a "reward center" of the brain, associated with positive emotion and feelings of affiliation. You also know this experientially, because it is part of the reason why it feels good to help people. Taking action to serve others in meaningful ways is also associated with increased production of endorphins, oxytocin, serotonin, and in some cases dopamine, in the giver (as well as the receiver), which potentiate the feel-good experience of compassion for (and service to) others.

In the field of OB/GYN, clinician compassion has profound implications for both the quality of patient care and healthcare outcomes. The role of compassion in this specialty is underscored by its unique emotional, physiological, and psychological benefits to patients, which are particularly critical given the potentially intimate nature of OB/GYN practice. In this section, we translate some of the scientific evidence for compassionate care into practical insights for OB/GYN practitioners. This evidence-based approach helps underscore the tangible benefits of integrating compassion into daily practice.

Compassionate care in OB/GYN can play a role in both maternal and fetal health. For example, compassion activates the parasympathetic nervous system (PNS), which has a calming effect. In contrast to activation of the sympathetic nervous system (i.e., "fight or flight" response), PNS activation results in lower heart rate and respiratory rate and blood pressure and increased heart rate variability, indicating greater cardiovascular homeostasis. These effects may be particularly beneficial during pregnancy, where maternal stress management may be considered an important factor.

In addition, research supports that compassionate care may reduce a person's experience of pain. Of course, compassion cannot eliminate pain entirely. However, numerous studies of experimentally induced pain in laboratories, as well as clinical studies, support that compassion, e.g., the touch of a trusted other, can reduce a person's experience of pain to an extent that can in fact be measured, at least in the context of a research study. That said, the clinical meaningfulness of the impact on pain may vary substantially from person to person and be context-dependent. We submit that, given the low "cost" of compassionate care and the potential benefits for patients, clinician compassion should be considered an integral component of treatment for all painful conditions or experiences.

The motivation for optimal self-care is another critical effect of compassionate care. Broadly, if a clinician cares deeply about patients, and their patients know it, they are more likely to take their medicine (i.e., medication adherence instead of non-adherence). They are also more likely to follow treatment recommendations and less likely to be lost to follow-up. One specific element of patient experience, knowing the patient "as a person," has been linked to sharply higher patient adherence to prescribed therapy among patients with a serious chronic condition. In OB/GYN, where patient education and proactive health management can be pivotal, compassion can encourage more active patient participation. Patients who perceive their caregivers as empathetic and supportive are more likely to engage in recommended self-care routines, follow medical advice, and access necessary health services. This engagement is essential for managing chronic conditions, optimizing pregnancy outcomes, and improving overall women's health across the lifespan.

Psychologically, compassion creates a supportive environment that can significantly impact symptoms of anxiety and depression. This support may be vital during times of emotional vulnerability such as pregnancy, infertility treatments, or postpartum periods. The mental health benefits also extend to better coping strategies during stressful procedures and transitions. Although we are not aware of any studies specifically on the impact of compassion on postpartum depression, numerous studies show that compassion is foundational to the therapeutic relationship for patients experiencing depression in general. Compassion from a clinician can have a moderate to large effect size on depression symptoms among patients suffering from depression. Specifically, compassion has been found to combat demoralization, which is a patient's depression about their depression, the hopeless belief that they are never going to get better. In this way, compassion can be a powerful restorer of hope.

Clinician compassion is also associated with high-quality healthcare. In healthcare environments where there is less caring, research supports that patients are less safe. Numerous studies have shown that when clinicians suffer from depersonalization, i.e., difficulty making personal connections with patients, the clinicians' risk of a major self-reported medical or surgical error is sharply higher. Although cause-and-effect cannot be established from the study designs in this research, a causal pathway is plausible on the grounds that disconnected and detached clinicians may be less meticulous about the quality of care that they provide, compared to fully engaged clinicians. This risk is supported by evidence that clinicians suffering from depersonalization are more likely to provide suboptimal care. That is, in the context of an anonymous research study, they admit "cutting corners" in patient care and deviating from what is considered "best practice."

When adverse outcomes do occur, abundant research supports that consistently compassionate care can also reduce the risk of a medical malpractice lawsuit. In fact, research supports that most medical malpractice claims do not actually involve malpractice, and most actual malpractice events do not result in a medical malpractice claim being filed. Research shows that a critical determinant of a patient's (or family's) decision to file a medical malpractice claim is the quality of the relationship with the involved clinician(s). We can distill the salient points of numerous studies down to this: When adverse outcomes occur (and adverse outcomes can occur despite technically excellent care), if patients believe you care about them and you were trying your best, a malpractice claim is much less likely. Conversely, if patients think you do not care, or they experienced a loss of dignity or respect in the care you provided, a medical malpractice claim is much more likely, even if the care you provided was technically sound. This is an important concept for all physicians to grasp as they begin their career, and it is especially important for OB/GYN, given the medical malpractice risks inherent in the specialty.

Strategies for Enhancing Compassion in Practice

To integrate compassion effectively, OB/GYN practitioners should focus on empathy, communication, and patient-centered care practices. Training in compassionate communication should be a cornerstone of medical education and continuing professional development. Workshops on empathetic listening, recognizing non-verbal cues, and managing emotional responses can equip practitioners with the skills needed to foster deeper patient relationships. Additionally, institutions should support environments that promote compassion, recognizing its impact on both patient and clinician well-being. It is important for health system leaders to realize that compassionate care is not merely a "nice to have"; rather, compassion is an integral component of high-quality healthcare that merits being an institutional imperative.

Importantly, there is ample research to support that clinicians can get better at compassion for patients. Research supports that adopting a growth mindset about compassion, i.e., the belief that compassion is a set of skills to be practiced and mastered rather than a trait that we are either born with or not, is a vital first step in improvement. Accordingly, clinicians need to believe (correctly) that they can in fact get better at compassion for patients, coupled with a desire to improve. A recent systematic review found that 75% of the published studies of compassion curricula for clinicians resulted in an increase in compassionate behaviors by clinicians, and this included studies assessing compassion from the patient perspective.

Overcoming Potential Barriers to Compassionate Care

The barriers to compassionate care in health systems are multifaceted, encompassing both systemic issues and personal challenges faced by healthcare providers. One significant barrier is the interruption of patients by physicians when patients are trying to communicate their concerns. Research supports that this occurs alarmingly early during consultations. For example, one study found that the mean elapsed time before a physician interrupts a patient when they are trying to state their main concern is only 11 s, despite patients typically needing only 29 s to communicate their concerns. Research also supports that this trend of premature interruption has worsened over time.

Another potential barrier may be an unintended consequence of the development of electronic medical records (EMRs), which, although designed to enhance documentation and patient safety, can distract healthcare providers from eye contact with patients during consultations. This is a risk to the quality of care because physicians may miss important emotional cues from patients. This is especially important in a field like OB/GYN, where patients often share highly personal and perhaps sensitive information. Thus, a lack of eye contact may impair the quality of care. Fortunately, new technologies are under development that leverage conversational, ambient, and generative artificial intelligence (AI) to "listen" to the clinical encounter and automate note creation, so that clinicians can focus on patients rather than focusing on a computer screen. In contrast to the first-generation EMRs without AI augmentation, it is expected that these new technologies will enhance the patient experience rather than detracting from it.

Time constraints also pose a significant barrier to compassionate care in the minds of many clinicians. Many healthcare providers believe they do not have enough time to provide compassionate care, reflecting a deeper systemic issue within the healthcare industry, where efficiency often takes precedence over human connection. However, the belief that we do not have time for compassion in clinical practice is not supported by the available evidence. The published data supports that compassion does not actually take much time at all. In fact, meaningful compassionate connections with patients can be established in a remarkably short amount of time, just 40 s according to a study published in the *Journal of Clinical Oncology*. Brief, genuine displays of compassion, such as a thoughtful question or a moment of attentive listening, can be deeply impactful to patients, communicating care and concern effectively without requiring lengthy time commitments. This approach is particularly valuable in fast-paced medical settings like OB/GYN, where time is a premium, but the need for compassionate care remains critical.

Effects of Compassionate Care on Clinicians

The available evidence in the scientific literature supports that compassionate care can have powerful beneficial effects for the giver, too. Conventional thinking in medical training in decades past, commonly communicated to students and trainees via the "hidden curriculum," was that physicians should not care "too much" about patients, because too much caring leads to burnout. Now, with the advent of numerous research studies, rather than opinion and anecdotes, we find compelling evidence for the opposite. In fact, according to a systematic review, 80% of the published studies find an *inverse* association between clinician compassion and burnout. One mechanism may be through deeper relationships that flow from compassionate care. Meaningful relationships with patients can build resilience to the inherent stresses of clinical practice. This is also true of deeper, more meaningful relationships with colleagues, coworkers, trainees, and all others in the healthcare environment. If we want to build resilience and resistance to burnout, an evidence-based approach would be to invest in relationships, and a foundational piece of these relationships is empathy and compassion for others. We do not hold out compassion as a solitary "antidote" to burnout in isolation, but rather a key ingredient to more meaningful relationships and all the associated benefits.

Conclusion

Incorporating the science of compassion into OB/GYN not only improves patient outcomes but enriches the caregiving process, making it more satisfying and sustainable. It builds a healthcare culture that values and prioritizes patient well-being, enhances professional satisfaction among healthcare providers, and constructs a more humane and effective healthcare system. Embracing compassion is not merely an ethical choice; it is a practical and scientifically sound approach that enhances patient experience, improves patient outcomes, and enriches the careers and lives of those who care for patients.

Further reading

Trzeciak S, Mazzarelli A. Compassionomics: the revolutionary scientific evidence that caring makes a difference. Huron Publishing; 2019.

Trzeciak S, Mazzarelli A. Wonder drug: 7 scientifically proven ways that serving others is the best medicine for yourself. St. Martin's Essentials; 2022.

Patel S, Pelletier-Bui A, Smith S, Roberts MB, Kilgannon H, Trzeciak S, Roberts BW. Curricula for empathy and compassion training in medical education: a systematic review. PLoS One. 2019;14(8):e0221412.

Trzeciak S, Roberts BW, Mazzarelli A. Compassionomics: hypothesis and experimental approach. Med Hypotheses. 2017;107:92–7.

Chapter 25
Working with Medical Students

Kristina Williams

Introduction

All physicians have been through the medical school process and can remember the stress and anxiety experienced during their clinical rotations. They can likely identify faculty they worked with who have had a significant impact on their training, whether positive or negative. As becoming a physician is an apprenticeship in many ways, teaching faculty immensely impact a young student physician's growth in all medical fields. Obstetrics and Gynecology (OBGYN) is a core clinical experience in most US medical schools. You may encounter medical students in their preclinical or clinical years, whether working in a community or an academic center. Indeed, if your institution is associated with a medical school, it is very likely that you will be asked or required to educate medical students. In the preclinical years, this may include lecturing students, leading case-based discussions, or allowing students to shadow you in the operating room, office, or on labor and delivery. During the clinical years, faculty are required to supervise students in their learning journey to see, evaluate, and manage patients.

Student Learning Goals

Students have impressionable minds and are often undifferentiated upon their first encounter with OBGYN. Not only is it essential to teach all students basic OBGYN topics, but a student's experience working within the OBGYN department tends to

K. Williams (✉)
Department of Obstetrics and Gynecology, Cooper Medical School of Rowan University and Cooper University Health Care, Camden, NJ, USA

A. Malik et al. (eds.), *An Obstetrician/Gynecologist's Path*,
https://doi.org/10.1007/978-3-031-87098-9_25

significantly impact the ability to recruit young minds into the field. It is essential to recognize that most students encountered during the core clinical OBGYN experience will choose something other than OBGYN as a field. According to AAMC data, only 6.6% of graduating students plan to pursue OBGYN as a career [1]. Since most medical students will not choose OBGYN as a field, the students you work with may exhibit a different passion for the field than you or a resident may have. Additionally, the learning goals of a core clinical year medical student will differ from those of a fourth-year student rotating on OBGYN or an OBGYN resident.

Clinical faculty at each medical school are responsible for defining learning objectives and required clinical encounters for their students. As such, each medical school will have a unique outline of what each student must learn and complete. If you are working with students, you should receive learning objectives from the student's institution. In general, core clerkship students should learn the basic concepts of OBGYN, emphasizing evaluation and diagnosis. At the end of their core clinical experience, they should develop the skills to take focused OBGYN histories, perform breast and pelvic exams, and discuss sensitive topics with patients. While being able to follow directions and being prepared are essential, core clerkship students do not need to develop surgical skills such as assisting, knot tying, and suturing. However, these skills should be taught so that students interested in pursuing surgical specialties can develop them during their advanced clinical rotations.

Student Experience

Being mindful of the student experience is essential when working with students as teaching faculty. Medical education is continuously evolving, and there is a much heavier emphasis on the student experience, as measured by the AAMC's Graduation Questionnaire (GQ). The GQ is an anonymous survey administered to all graduating US M.D. students. From 2019 to 2023, annual data shows that the overall quality of the OBGYN clerkship is rated as "good" or "excellent" by 77–78% of graduating medical students, in comparison to the internal medicine clerkship at 91–92% and even the surgery clerkship at 81–83% [1]. It is essential to pay attention to GQ data as the LCME uses it to assess schools and make re-accreditation decisions. More importantly, to improve the student experience on OBGYN, we must understand why OBGYN is rated lower by students compared to other specialties. Numerous reasons have been suggested, including long work hours, decreased hands-on experience, accessibility of faculty, ineffective teaching by residents/fellows, and mistreatment, which is prevalent within the OBGYN clerkship [2, 3]. According to 2023 GQ data, for students who reported experiencing or witnessing mistreatment during their medical school experience, approximately 31% reported that this occurred during their OBGYN clerkship [1]. It is the job of the administration and core clerkship leadership to address these issues, but individual teaching faculty play a substantial role in the student experience.

Creating a Positive Learning Environment

As teaching faculty and leader of the clinical team, it is your responsibility to create a positive learning and working environment. This is done by creating an atmosphere of psychological safety, defined as "a shared belief that the team is safe for interpersonal risk-taking" [4]. An atmosphere of psychological safety will allow all team members, including learners, to ask questions and share thoughts without fear of negative consequences. Setting the stage, inviting participation, and showing genuine appreciation are the critical steps in creating psychological safety within the team learning environment [5]. In OBGYN, an atmosphere of psychological safety will help students release some of their preconceptions and anxiety regarding their imminent clinical experience in OBGYN and better allow students the ability to engage and take initiative.

The OBGYN service can be intimidating for medical students. It is fast-paced, and students tend to need help finding their place. Setting the stage will help them to know what is expected of them. In doing so, asking students about their learning goals will allow the student to feel that you are invested in their learning. Setting learning goals and expectations will help you and the student work together effectively. Students deserve the same respect you would give any other colleague when working with them. They have a better experience working with educators who show respect, including acknowledging students, learning their names, and treating others respectfully [6].

One well-known expectation for a student in the OBGYN clinical experience is that it is their responsibility to walk into the room and introduce themselves to everyone. Better yet, they are sometimes told to find the attending and introduce themselves to that person. Placing this responsibility on the student can create an unwelcoming environment. They end up being ignored if they are not outgoing enough to complete this task reliably. As simple as it sounds, introducing yourself to students and getting to know their names goes a long way in showing respect toward students and creating a welcoming environment. Additionally, students will perceive you as approachable and feel less nervous while working with you. They will feel more comfortable contributing to patient care and are more likely to be engaged overall. Additionally, it is important to acknowledge students for their contributions to the team. Thanking them for assisting in surgery, completing a task for a patient, or asking a thoughtful question will provide positive reinforcement and help the student continue to engage.

While building a positive learning environment, it is crucial to avoid setbacks that will cause breakdowns in psychological safety. The OBGYN service can be acute, causing stress and tension within the team, and learners may make mistakes in this setting. It is essential not to yell or berate a student. If they do something incorrectly, it is a learning experience for them. Do not disengage with them. Let them know what they did incorrectly and move on from the situation. You should continue to include them in the clinical activity. Doing so does not mean allowing them to perform a task or procedure that they did not prepare for, but you should always continue to teach every student, regardless of their preparedness. As a role model to learners, you should ALWAYS be the bigger person.

Excessive work hours can also impact the clinical working environment. Long work hours can cause fatigue and negatively impact student performance, thus leading to a poor experience. The days when medical student apprenticeships must mimic the work hours of an OBGYN resident are long gone. While students understand that their clinical years will be tough, they tend to dislike staying late and being present for calls if they are not needed. For example, a medical student may feel it less beneficial to continue to observe a surgery past the end of the workday (i.e., 5 pm), primarily because they still need to put time into studying during their clerkship. Students can learn the basics of OBGYN and participate in the necessary clinical experiences without working excessive hours. Thus, as clinical faculty, it is important to be mindful of the work hours you ask of a student. If there are no additional clinical experiences for the student to participate in, it is best to allow them to use their time as they would like.

Being an Effective Educator

One of the most challenging and underrated aspects of being an OBGYN educator is that you must develop skills to teach in many different settings to succeed. While an emergency medicine or a family medicine physician teaches their specialty in one setting, the OBGYN educator will be responsible for educating in the ambulatory setting, the operating room, the labor floor (i.e., ICU level care), in triages, and through inpatient medicine as a consulting physician. The diversity that the OBYGN physician loves so much about the specialty can sometimes be the biggest challenge when teaching someone what they need to know in OBGYN. For example, you may find it easy to teach a student in the ambulatory setting but have not yet developed the skills necessary to teach in the OR setting. Students will find this frustrating because, in specific settings, they may feel that they have not had an adequate learning experience or have not been challenged enough to be evaluated.

Continual faculty development is necessary to be a clinical educator. The five-step "microskills" model of clinical teaching is a well-known primer for teaching for clinical faculty [7]. In addition to this resource, the Association of Professors of Obstetrics and Gynecology (APGO), the educational society within OBGYN, publishes an effective preceptor series, which can be found at www.apgo.org/resources. The series provides practical tools for OBGYN clinical faculty to develop the skills necessary to educate and evaluate students. The series comprises 12 easy-to-read PDFs that provide guidance on topics such as teaching in an ambulatory setting, teaching in the OR, preparing for learners, and much more. This is an excellent starting place for any OBGYN teaching faculty interested in becoming a better educator. The guides break down the information to make the task of teaching in multiple settings seem much less daunting.

Balancing Clinical Duties with Educating Medical Students

Finding the time to teach medical students while providing excellent patient care can be very challenging for a busy clinician. When working with learners, completing clinical tasks will take longer. Some institutions will give protected teaching time to faculty required to teach students. However, for most clinical faculty, expectations of teaching students (and residents) are part of the job description. Again, OBGYN clinical faculty teach in many settings—the operating room, the office, the inpatient setting, and the labor and delivery floor. The biggest challenge to integrating students is that the approach will differ in each setting. What should be avoided in balancing clinical care and student education is consistently placing students into a shadowing role and ignoring medical students.

While reports of mistreatment of medical students are known to be higher in surgical specialties, another issue that students face is neglect, which creates a suboptimal learning environment. Neglect can quickly happen on a busy OBGYN service. Imagine being on a labor floor on a busy day. You are going from room to room, putting out small fires. When focusing primarily on patient care, it is easy to forget that a student is present. The student would have loved to be part of the completed tasks, but because you have completed your clinical tasks without the student, they now may assume that you purposefully left them out of the clinical care. Therefore, they step back and no longer volunteer for additional clinical experiences because they feel you do not want them around.

The patient is always the priority in the clinical setting, and the students must understand that. However, clinical educators must learn to balance patient care and student education. Ideally, when setting the stage for students, you will permit them to take initiative. Creating specific tasks, goals, and expectations for the student will allow the student to function throughout the day without being micromanaged, potentially removing some of the stress of needing to worry about the student. If you are working on a busy labor floor, permitting a student to follow you, even if you do not expressly say so, allows them to feel comfortable stepping up. In the office, setting a goal of how many patients you want the student to see and evaluate gives the student an attainable goal. By setting this goal, they are less likely to feel neglected if you start seeing patients without them because they are working on reviewing their own patient's charts or writing notes. In an acute setting, like an emergency cesarean section, you may be so focused on the patient that you will forget the student is there. However, once the acuity dies down, you should be mindful to include the student by inviting them to scrub at the end of the procedure and/or debriefing the situation.

There is no one-size-fits-all method for balancing patient care and student education; techniques will depend on your teaching style. Experience will help you identify ways to avoid student neglect and to promote the student from the shadowing role while still effectively managing an office session or inpatient floor.

Conclusion

When working with medical students as OBGYN clinical faculty, it is vital to ensure a positive learning environment, which includes setting student expectations, showing respect and inclusivity, and avoiding neglect. Being an effective clinical educator is challenging, given the diversity of clinical settings in which OBGYN faculty work. You must work toward finding a balance between student education and clinical care; this will allow you to enjoy the rewarding aspects of teaching students clinical OBGYN.

References

1. AAMC. 2023 GQ all schools summary report. 2023. www.aamc.org/gq.
2. Burke WM, Williams JA, Fenner DE, Hammoud MM. The obstetrics and gynecology clerkship: building a better model from past experience. Am J Obstet Gynecol. 2004;191(5):1772–6. https://doi.org/10.1016/j.ajog.2004.07.061.
3. Pradhan A, Page-Ramsey S, Buery-Joyner SD, Craig LB, Dalrymple JL, Forstein DA, Graziano S, Hampton BS, Hopkins L, McKenzie M, Wolf A, Abbott JF. Undergraduate obstetrics and gynecology medical education: why are we underrated and underappreciated? Am J Obstet Gynecol. 2016;214(3):345–7. https://doi.org/10.1016/j.ajog.2015.10.915.
4. Edmondson A. Psychological safety and learning behavior in work teams. Adm Sci Q. 1999;44(2):350–83. https://doi.org/10.2307/2666999.
5. McClintock AH, Fainstad T. Growth, engagement, and belonging in the clinical learning environment: the role of psychological safety and the work ahead. J Gen Intern Med. 2022;37(9):2291–6. https://doi.org/10.1007/s11606-022-07493-6.
6. Dickinson KJ, Bass BL, Pei KY. Medical students' perception of what embodies an effective surgeon educator. Am J Surg. 2022;223(1):64–70. https://doi.org/10.1016/j.amjsurg.2021.07.019.
7. Neher JO, Gordon KC, Meyer B, Stevens N. A five-step "microskills" model of clinical teaching. J Am Board Fam Pract. 1992;5(4):419–24. https://www.ncbi.nlm.nih.gov/pubmed/1496899.

Chapter 26
Interactions with Residents

Kyle Le and Yon Sook Kim

Setting Expectations and Communication

Clearly outline your expectations regarding patient care, documentation, and professionalism. Establishing open lines of communication with residents is crucial. Effective communication will ensure the resident and the attending understand expectations and responsibilities. Be approachable and supportive, and encourage residents to share their concerns, ask questions, and seek guidance regarding patient management. Setting clear expectations will establish a foundation for effective teamwork.

Provide Constructive Feedback

An essential aspect of education is giving and receiving feedback, which is crucial for growth and improvement. Before giving feedback, it is vital to ask the resident to reflect on their performance and self-assess. Provide feedback on clinical skills, communication, and professionalism. There are generally two types of feedback: informal and formal. Informal feedback is given during a procedure or walking

K. Le
Reproductive Endocrinology and Infertility, Jones Institute at Old Dominion University, Norfolk, VA, USA

Department of Obstetrics and Gynecology, Cooper Medical School of Rowan University and Cooper University Health Care, Camden, NJ, USA

Y. S. Kim (✉)
Department of Obstetrics and Gynecology, Cooper Medical School of Rowan University and Cooper University Health Care, Camden, NJ, USA

A. Malik et al. (eds.), *An Obstetrician/Gynecologist's Path*,
https://doi.org/10.1007/978-3-031-87098-9_26

between patient rooms during the clinic. This type of feedback allows the resident to adjust immediately during a procedure (i.e., in how they are holding their needle or tying their knots) or in patient interactions and other clinical duties such as writing notes or placing orders. Informal feedback is more casual and is generally quick and short.

On the other hand, formal feedback is typically in a written form, more structured, planned, and scheduled. Complete feedback promptly, objectively, and constructively. It should always be in a private setting. Feedback should focus on specific areas or behaviors to improve and be actionable to address the issues so that the residents receiving that feedback can find ways to improve.

After receiving feedback, the residents may have questions regarding why they received the feedback that they did; therefore, documentation of specific examples is helpful. Detailed examples help the resident better understand and contextualize their input. It is also important to remember that receiving and accepting feedback may take time. Feedback should be honest and direct but also gentle. The attending may need to alter how feedback is provided depending on the personality of the person receiving it so that it is received more positively. It may take some time to develop your style of giving feedback, and you may want to solicit your own feedback or have a more experienced mentor observe you in order to help you improve.

Encourage Independence

Residents learn by observing and then doing. Recognize that OB/GYN residents are at different stages of their training. There is a tremendous amount of information to comprehend, especially during the intern year, and a steep learning curve exists. Repetition of performing clinical duties and techniques in the operating room allows for solidification of fundamental skills. One example of how to promote independence may be prompting a resident to formulate an assessment and plan and, for example, asking the resident for their labor induction plan at the end of their triage patient presentation. Another way is to discuss with the resident what instruments and surgical tools they desire in the operating room. For example, what instruments does the resident want to use to enter the abdomen during laparoscopy? If there is a disagreement with the resident's plan, then a discussion on the reasoning may be undertaken so that they may better understand. Encouraging the residents to participate actively in patient care and decision-making will allow them to develop their skills and gain confidence within a supportive environment. Remember that learners have different learning styles, backgrounds, and confidence levels.

As an attending, it is essential to know that residents in their first 2 years will require more supervision than residents in their third and fourth years. The third- and fourth-year residents are in the developmental stages of formulating their practice styles, clinically and surgically, and will require more independence than junior residents. Furthermore, patient cases that are more medically complex will require increased vigilance and supervision from the attending. Though necessary to review on a case-by-case basis, it will benefit the resident to have autonomy and independence whenever possible. As a new attending, it will be a balance between allowing residents freedom and preventing patient harm.

Teaching in the Operating Room

Surgical attendings must balance their responsibilities: they must preserve patient safety and allow future surgeons to function as the primary surgeons to learn and gain confidence. Residents must have the chance to be independent and meaningfully learn during a case. At the same time, hospitals will track the total time of a surgeon's cases—shorter cases are less costly, and patient outcomes worsen if surgeries take longer [1, 2]. Overall, patient safety should always take priority over the teaching of residents. However, when opportunities arise, residents should be allowed to learn in a safe setting.

Informal feedback can be given to residents during the procedure to guide them in the right direction. Urging residents to slow down with verbal cues in crucial procedure steps, such as the skeletonizing and ligating of uterine vessels in a hysterectomy, is vital. Residents should be encouraged to speed up for patient safety in other portions of the case—as more prolonged cases increase patient complications. The residents may ask questions throughout the procedure to better understand the attending's thought processes as they operate. Furthermore, you can make suggestions to improve their surgical technique, such as how they suture or perform electrocautery. Many learners retain the steps of a procedure if they understand the reasoning behind a particular step. As the attending surgeon, it is crucial to explain to the resident why one is acting in a specific manner or order—at times, there may not be a significant reason other than personal preference, but knowing the reason may help the resident learn and develop their style in the operating room. It is also essential to be consistent in how you perform each surgical case. Residents will remember the particular style of how the attending likes to operate and perform the procedure similarly to be more efficient.

If there is a bad outcome after a procedure, debriefing with the resident regarding what may have gone awry can be beneficial. The debriefing may be more formal, but it can also be informal. It may benefit the attending surgeon and resident, as well as future patients, to understand why a surgical complication occurred and help prevent future errors.

Mentorship

Respect is the foundation of any successful mentor-resident relationship, and mentorship is crucial to medical education. It can be rewarding to help shape the careers of the next generation of OBGYN providers. Mentorship can also be formal or informal in how the relationship forms. Some residency programs will have a mentorship program in which the resident will be assigned a mentor or choose a mentor based on shared interests or career goals. Other programs may have an informal process that happens more organically. There are multiple mentoring models, including dyadic, multiple, apprenticeship, and team [3]. The dyadic mentorship model is the traditional mentoring model with a one-on-one relationship between a mentor and a mentee, and this is the most common type of mentoring model [3]. The multiple mentorship model is when a mentee is mentored by multiple mentors in different areas of expertise [3].

The mentee should define goals at the beginning of the relationship. The mentor takes on a more generous role in that they may advocate for and support their mentee in achieving their established goals. Completing the set goals will take time, and the process will require the mentee's persistence and the mentor's patience. An essential aspect of the relationship is that the mentor should be honest with the mentee in giving feedback. It is a more favorable scenario for the mentee to receive feedback from someone they trust and have a working relationship with, such as a mentor. Mentors should also be able to alter their interpersonal communication style depending on the mentee.

Regarding benefits for the mentor in this relationship, the mentee may expose the mentor to novel ideas and opportunities or help the mentor relearn material. For example, if research is the mentee's interest, the mentee may propose novel research ideas to the mentor, who can guide the further development of the research project. Lastly, a good mentor should care about the mentee's professional and personal growth. It is rewarding to help a mentee succeed in their career goals and, in the process, develop a long-term personal relationship with the mentee, who will eventually become a peer in the field.

On the other hand, as a new attending, finding your mentors is also crucial. Mentors should have the expertise or quality that you are looking for. For example, if your interest is research, finding a mentor with expertise in grant writing, statistics, and manuscript writing is essential. Mentorship is a crucial aspect of growth in the medical field for all people at different stages of their careers.

Lifelong Learner

Staying up to date will increase your confidence when working with residents. Teaching your residents the latest guidelines will positively impact your performance and your interactions with residents. Residents respect attendings who regularly update their knowledge and skills and do not say, "That is how I have always done it." Keeping up to date will also promote the importance of practicing evidence-based medicine. Encourage the residents to appraise the literature critically and base their clinical decisions on the best available evidence. Be open to learning from your residents also. You will learn something new every day. Read the current literature, attend educational conferences, and share your knowledge with the team.

Conclusion

Working with residents is a rewarding experience. Creating a positive and collaborative working relationship conducive to everyone's professional growth is essential, enhancing the overall patient care experience. Lead by example and serve as a role model for communication skills, professionalism, and exceptional patient care. Treat residents with kindness, fairness, and respect, and they will do the same to you.

References

1. Jackson T, Wannares J, Lancaster R, et al. Does speed matter? The impact of operative time on outcome in laparoscopy. Surg Endo. 2011;25:2288–95.
2. Sutkin G, Littleton E, Kanter S. Maintaining operative efficiency while allowing sufficient time for residents to learn. Am J Surg. 2019;218:211–7.
3. Henry-Noel N, Bishop M, Gwede C, et al. Mentorship in medicine and other health professions. J Cancer Edu. 2019;34:629–37.

Chapter 27
Interactions with Nursing

Rori Dajao and Laura Brown

Interactions with Nursing

There is nothing braver than a Chief Resident. You are (seemingly) at the top of your knowledge and skills. There are no situations that you are unable to handle. Attendings prefer your help over other residents. Then, your first attending call comes, and you realize that now your name is going to be at the bottom of every delivery note, progress note, and operative note for the next 12–24 h. Moreover, if you work with residents, you realize that you will have to look over them to ensure that everything is done safely! You are the safety net for the Brave Chief Resident. This sudden realization can be anxiety inducing. We were speaking about this anxiety as we were preparing for this chapter:

Dr. Dajao: My anxiety was through the roof on my first night on call. After getting sign out for the shift, one of the first places I went to for comfort was the nurses' station. The nurses there had all just witnessed my transformation from PGY-1 to a brand new PGY-5 (aka attending) but also supported and guided many before me on the same journey.

Laura, RN: As a labor and delivery nurse for 13 years, I witnessed many physicians navigating their first shifts as attendings. I also have joined many physicians for first emergent cesarean section, first shoulder dystocia, first time identifying a fetal loss and countless other trying situations. I very quickly realized that to navigate through these situations, whether it is your first time or your one hundredth time, you need to be able to trust, communicate with and lean on those around you:

R. Dajao
Department of Obstetrics and Gynecology, Cooper Medical School of Rowan University and Cooper University Health Care, Camden, NJ, USA

L. Brown (✉)
Cooper University Health Care, Camden, NJ, USA

A. Malik et al. (eds.), *An Obstetrician/Gynecologist's Path*,
https://doi.org/10.1007/978-3-031-87098-9_27

not only clinically but also emotionally. The specialty we chose is not always easy, and the strength of your team is critical to success.

Dr. Dajao: Agreed. It's usually a happy time on Labor and Delivery which makes sad times absolutely tragic. So having a team that you are comfortable with is a big plus. This wasn't just true for me because I stayed at a place where I had trained. Many of my colleagues stated that senior nurses were a big help in easing the transition to being a new attending and being at a new hospital.

Nurses are your eyes and ears. They will tell you how your patient is doing, not only with objective data such as vital signs but also with subjective criteria such as how your patients (and their support people) are coping with the labor process. It is incumbent on you to take their information and insight seriously and act on it. The best way to ensure that this happens can be distilled into a single word: Communicate!

Labor and Delivery is an intense, high-stake clinical environment and communication issues are major root causes of many patient safety events. If communication is timely, clear, respectful, and actionable, it creates a sense of team that increases camaraderie, ownership, accountability, and therefore safety. It is important to remember that in healthcare, the vast majority of people come to work to help patients. Therefore, in a clinically tenuous situation, keep this in mind when communicating with the nurses on your team. They want to help the patient, just as you do, and active collaboration with them is the best way to accomplish this. Keep them involved in discussions with the patient so that everyone is on the same page. Keep the whole team involved and updated when you have multiple complex patients whom you are dealing with. If you don't agree with a suggestion from them or anyone else on the team, provide clinical reasoning as to why you are proceeding with your plan of care. Use accepted guidelines and shared terminology, again to ensure that the entire team is on the same page. For example, "I'm fine with the tracing, start the pito," has a different tone than "The tracing is Category 2; there are intermittent late decelerations, but on the other hand, there are accelerations and moderate variability, so I think we can start the pitocin, what are your concerns?"

Despite our best efforts, conflict within the team is inevitable. How we handle this conflict is critical for creating and maintaining a team that operates safely and effectively under high-stress, high-stakes situations. Professional, respectful, and effective communication creates an environment where ALL healthcare providers feel empowered to raise concerns and advocate for patients. Conflict management is complicated by many factors. Everyone has a different comfort level when dealing with conflict. No two individuals handle conflict in the same way. The nature of the environment in which we practice often requires conflict to be addressed under ticking clocks and time constraints. This stressful setting often causes individuals to respond to conflict in a manner that may not be consistent with their personality. Is this a lot to consider while simultaneously working to safely manage complicated clinical situations? The answer is profoundly "YES." For this reason, despite good intentions, professional, respectful resolution of conflict often falls to the bottom of the priority list.

Another critical point to consider when entering the realm of attending is that your response to conflict will inevitably be not only noticed but also mirrored.

Residents, nurses, and fellow attendings consider your behavior when they decide how to handle these complicated situations. They will look for YOU to guide them through these uncomfortable, unfamiliar situations. The pressure is on but not to worry, it is possible to navigate these situations safely and respectfully.

When encountering conflict within the team, the most important thing to remember is that we are a team of healthcare professionals working TOGETHER to ensure the safety and well-being of our patients. Each discipline offers the expertise that the team needs to function safely and effectively. If you consistently and genuinely view the team in this way, you are off to a great start.

When communicating with a team, it is important to use shared terminology. For example, our personal favorite is the Huddle [1]. Our team uses the word "Huddle" to call an in-person meeting of the entire team of healthcare providers caring for a patient (or group of patients) at any given time. It is used when any member of the team has a concern with or needs clarification of a plan of care. Simply using this shared terminology allows for concise, clear communication and helps to eliminate misconceptions. Note that the consistent use of these terms does not happen overnight. As with any change in culture, it may take a while but eventually the team will embrace the ease that they bring to communication.

For everyone on the team to feel comfortable moving forward through a conflict, it is important that every team member express their concerns and feel heard. When one can express concerns in a safe space and be met with consideration and respect, a sense of trust is built within the team. Trust is crucial for a team to operate safely and effectively. Each time the team moves through conflict in a respectful and professional way, the team as a whole becomes stronger.

On that note, it is important to acknowledge that the team will not work through conflict flawlessly every time. It is inevitable that tempers will be lost, and voices and opinions will go unheard. In addition, yes, it is possible to safely care for patients while being wildly unprofessional—the patient outcome can be 100% safe in that single instance. However, acting unprofessionally repeatedly can slowly but surely erode team dynamics, causing many more far-reaching, big picture problems. An unsafe environment is created not only for patients but also for the team itself. Each time these behaviors occur, a little bit of trust is lost within the team. Repeated unprofessional behavior can therefore result in an unprofessional unit culture that can take years to correct. To avoid this, modeling professional, respectful behavior is crucial to creating and maintaining a safe and professional culture. In addition, be sure to acknowledge when the team falls short when moving through conflict, learn from that, and commit to doing better next time.

One final note to keep in mind is that conflict often presents an opportunity for learning among disciplines. Conflict can create a setting where healthcare providers can come together to share experience and knowledge with one another to improve care for a patient. Disagreements may be an opportunity to share the newest research study and/or oldest provider experience, enhancing every team member's knowledge base. Moreover, clinical knowledge is not the only thing being shared. Effective, respectful, and professional behavior is modeled. By patiently practicing effective conflict resolution, team members can model and share communication tools that can be applied during future interactions. In the end, the entire team benefits, and everyone gets through the shift ready to take on the next.

Reference

1. https://urldefense.com/v3/__https://www.ahrq.gov/teamstepps-program/curriculum/team/tools/huddle.html__;!!NLFGqXoFfo8MMQ!vUnN5oVNAI6iLw7a%2D%2DIy0g90LGh-TjGlvi1YM5ak2tMoTS3ly0Tz4qdd5f5VmV7QPZ7nhtVdJ8b4sLh6t3f14eleQijjWLdpaX63tuHMv$.

Chapter 28
First Call with Your First Emergent Case as an Attending

Amanda Malik

In the world of ob/gyn, the very thing that attracted many of us to the field can become the thing that intimidates us the most: the unpredictability and variability of call. As a medical student, I remember the exhilarating rush of a precipitous delivery, an OB alert to the helipad, or Level 0 case to the OR. As a resident, I developed the skills and confidence to address these urgent issues, and during my chief year often had the feeling of "*I got this*;" backed, of course, by knowing there was always an attending over my shoulder or across the table.

As an attending, you may find your mindset shifts. First, you are not a "resident" of the hospital anymore; unless you go right to a laborist or hospitalist position, it is likely you will find yourself spending much less time on Labor and Delivery or responding to emergency pages than you did before. Instead of doing emergent hospital work day in and day out, it is likely that you will spend much less time dealing with acute emergencies. Instead, they will come during call shifts. In the world of obstetrics and gynecology, these sometimes are predictable—the ruptured ectopic in a patient who had previously refused methotrexate, or the shoulder dystocia with a suspected macrosomic fetus—but often, they are not.

During one of my own first call shifts, I was covering a preterm C-section of diamniotic-dichorionic twins in a patient who had worsening preeclampsia with severe features. We expected somewhat of a difficult extraction, as one of the twins was in a transverse position. Luckily, that went smoothly. However, when the residents I was working with attempted to extract the placentas, only one of them came—I placed one hand inside the uterus to feel the plane, quickly realized that there wasn't one, and that the C-section was about to become a hysterectomy. A few days into my role as attending, I found myself about to do an unplanned C-hyst.

A. Malik (✉)
Department of Obstetrics and Gynecology, Cooper Medical School of Rowan University and Cooper University Health Care, Camden, NJ, USA
e-mail: Malik-Amanda@cooperhealth.edu

A. Malik et al. (eds.), *An Obstetrician/Gynecologist's Path*,
https://doi.org/10.1007/978-3-031-87098-9_28

A few things helped to make the case go smoothly. First, I made a decision rapidly and began acting on it. For emergent cases, time is of the essence, and I recalled from experience that shredding the placenta or waiting too long to start the hysterectomy would result in elevated blood loss. Second, while the resident team began closing the hysterotomy, I took a minute to think through my plan, including how I should allocate team members. This was a case where I felt it best for myself and the chief resident to operate together, while the junior resident stayed to assist. Third, I had the circulating nurse call for backup—if there wasn't another attending immediately available, at least they would know what was going on and could help if I really got into trouble. The adrenaline rush of the unexpected course of surgery kept me focused on the case at hand and the necessary next steps. With a bit of luck, an excellent chief resident, and a guest appearance by one of my colleagues who came to check in, the case went well. Still, I found myself second guessing the decision to proceed with a hysterectomy. It wasn't until the pathology report came back, confirming a placenta accreta, that I felt some relief and confidence—I *did* know what I was doing!

It is very likely that within your own first few days, weeks, or months of work as an attending, you will find yourself with an emergent case. Culturally we joke about the luck of a first year attending, but in reality, emergencies are part of the field of ob/gyn. When you do, it can help to "fake it till you make it." Confidently making a decision on your course of action and allowing your training to balance your adrenaline can help you provide the excellent care you are capable of, no matter the situation.

When the time comes, remember; take a deep breath. Rely on your training. Phone a friend when necessary. You've got this!

Chapter 29
How to Be Smart with Case Selection

Peter J. Chen

Introduction

The transition from a resident to becoming an attending is exhilarating but at the same time can also be difficult. In the beginning, scheduling gynecologic cases will involve many decisions, big and small. They may include tasks you've never had to do as a resident, such as providing case preference cards, attesting for correct pre-op checklists, and confirming the availability of appropriate assistants and surgical teams. These decisions are now yours to make. As the captain of the ship, the responsibility for making sure a patient comes out of surgery safely is now yours.

For a gynecological surgeon, complications resulting from non-cancer gynecologic surgery are always anticipated but rarely expected to happen. When complications do happen, they do not only cause patients to suffer, but they also cause emotional distress to the surgeon, regardless of years of experience in the operating room.

Careful preoperative planning for elective cases is one way you can help reduce the risk of complications and improve patient safety while still establishing your scope of practice. One of the first decisions you must make for yourself when out in practice is to make appropriate selection for cases.

P. J. Chen (✉)
Department of Obstetrics and Gynecology, Cooper Medical School of Rowan University and Cooper University Health Care, Camden, NJ, USA
e-mail: chen-peter@cooperhealth.edu

A. Malik et al. (eds.), *An Obstetrician/Gynecologist's Path*,
https://doi.org/10.1007/978-3-031-87098-9_29

Shaping Your Practice

When considering case selection, you will need to take into account practice patterns as well as the details of an individual case. What cases you perform will likely shape the perceptions about the work you do and eventually define your practice. You may define the scope of your work by making a list of procedures you want to be doing, along with a list of procedures you are qualified to perform and willing to do [1]. This is often influenced by the number of surgeons in the area of your practice who are dedicated to performing the same type of procedures on your list. It is better not to keep your list too narrow in the beginning while you are building a practice. You will establish yourself as a "go-to" gynecologic surgeon if you are able to accept referrals quickly and provide a wide range of surgical services to the patients referred to you.

Primum non Nocere

The phrase "first, do no harm" should continue to be a guiding principle in your practice. Once you have decided what your practice will look like in a general sense, you will be faced with decisions regarding individual case selection. Within the scope of your practice, there may be specific procedures you choose to avoid at first. You must carefully consider the resources available to you and determine whether they are adequate to perform certain cases [2]. If you are not practicing in a hospital with 24/7 subspecialties where intraoperative surgical consults are readily available, scheduling a complicated endometriosis case may not be a wise decision. Whether you have partners who perform the same procedures and are qualified to manage some of your patients is another factor to consider. It might be very difficult to give up some surgeries that you have worked hard learning during residency, but performing them without appropriate support will be even more difficult. If you are lucky enough to have an experienced partner who can help, keep the case. You can always continue to learn from them.

Individual patients will present their own unique challenges. It is acceptable and smart to defer extremely difficult cases to a more experienced surgeon as you start off. It is worse for the patient and your confidence to start with difficult cases you weren't quite ready for. If you are trying to build up your laparoscopy routines, you may want to hold off on scheduling a laparoscopic hysterectomy for a patient with a 16-week size fibroid uterus and 4 prior cesarean sections on day one. As time goes on, you will have the confidence and experience to tackle the most difficult surgical problems. It is a good idea to successfully complete as many straightforward cases as possible to establish your routine in the operating room as a new attending.

Be judicious about choosing the appropriate route of surgery [3]. In the age of minimally invasive surgery for just about anything, it is easy to forget that not every patient is a laparoscopic candidate. Sometimes trying to do too much laparoscopically or sticking with it too long can create more hardships. For example, while minimally invasive hysterectomy is the preferred option for some patients, open abdominal hysterectomy may be necessary and supported by *ACOG* when the vaginal or laparoscopic approach is not appropriate to manage the patient's clinical situation, when facilities cannot support less invasive surgical approaches, or when an attempt at a minimally invasive route to hysterectomy fails intraoperatively. If the case calls for converting to open, convert early. If the case calls for doing it open from the start, do it open.

Conclusion

Appropriate case selection requires one to exercise good common sense. Having the courage to accept self-limitations and the knowledge of the resources that are available to the surgeon is part of the fundamentals to good surgical outcomes. This is not only true in the beginning, but will continue to serve you well later in your career. Make decisions with the patients in mind. Do that as you are forging a new path in your career and your practice will grow with you.

References

1. Yoon-Flannery K, et al. A surgeon's path. What to expect after a general surgery residency. Cham, Switzerland: Springer; 2018.
2. ACOG Committee Opinion, No 674, September 2016. Guiding principles for privileging of innovative procedures in gynecologic surgery.
3. ACOG Committee Opinion, No 701, June 2017, reaffirmed 2021. Choosing the route of hysterectomy for benign disease.

Chapter 30
Avoiding Disaster in the Operating Room

Paul S. Zamostien

Introduction

Leaving the relative safety of a residency or fellowship and establishing oneself in a full-time practice situation can be a daunting prospect for most trainees. Over my years of supervising residents, a huge number have come to me as they neared graduation expressing similar questions.

"What if I do not have experience or knowledge of a particular problem or procedure?"

"What do I do if I encounter a surgical dilemma or complication that I have never previously handled alone?"

Most young physicians do have the requisite knowledge and judgment to avoid disaster in the operating room but have never had to exercise the necessary steps to do this because they may not have had to—yet. I recall an incident where a senior resident was unable to extract a baby during a cesarean delivery and turned the responsibility over to me. After the case, he asked how I was able to complete the delivery when he had been unable to accomplish the task. I answered that I was successful because I had to be. I had no one to ask for help and had to do whatever was necessary to elevate the fetal head from the uterus, while he had me available once he had difficulty.

With proper preparation and approach to your surgical cases, disaster can be avoided.

To try to avoid operating room disasters, we can turn to some axioms—self-evident truths that require no proof—and their corollaries—obvious deductions or easily drawn conclusions—to these axioms.

P. S. Zamostien (✉)
Planned Parenthood Southeastern Pennsylvania, Philadelphia, PA, USA

A. Malik et al. (eds.), *An Obstetrician/Gynecologist's Path*,
https://doi.org/10.1007/978-3-031-87098-9_30

Be Prepared

Benjamin Franklin wrote, "By failing to prepare, you're preparing to fail." Preparing for surgery starts with reviewing your history and physical findings as well as lab data and imaging studies in a logical, progressive manner and mentally reviewing the planned procedure. Go over the basic steps of the surgery and consider what instruments you may need to have available. Remember that your new hospital may not have a particular instrument that you used regularly in your training. Making a list of instruments that you have used in your training may be a worthwhile task before leaving for your new destination.

Make Your Patient Feel Like a VIP

It is not always an easy thing to do, but you should strive to make every one of your patients feel as if she is your most important patient. The time you take to explain the patient's diagnosis and planned procedure is crucial. Make it known to her that you do not want her to leave the pre-operative discussion with any questions and that if she does leave with unanswered questions, you want the cause to be her not asking the question rather than your not adequately answering it. Consent forms can be scary sounding, but conveying that stuff happens is important and trying to put these possible negative outcomes into proper perspective is essential.

Not every doctor can be the smartest or the finest surgeon, but everyone can give a damn! Make sure that your patient knows that you care about giving her the best possible outcome to the upcoming procedure.

Know Your Surgical Anatomy

This is the best way to stay out of trouble. Occasionally reviewing this can only make you a better surgeon.

Identify a Mentor or Mentors

There will come a time when you need to run a case by someone before you get to the operating room. You may need to review your findings and surgical plans with someone to confirm your impressions and decisions. You can reach out to one of your previous attendings, or even better, find people at your new hospital whose judgment you respect. It never hurts to bounce your ideas off of another respected clinician. They will be glad to discuss your case with you, make you feel better about your plans, and as an extra bonus, it will most likely make their day too.

You may need these same people to come to your aid intra-operatively if you run into trouble. This mentor could be one of your practice associates, a subspecialist, or simply someone whose judgment and surgical skills have impressed you.

Follow the Rules

From operating with multiple attending physicians, you have undoubtedly seen and heard many surgical "rules" to help you stay out of trouble. You have seen great surgeons that have taught you by example and by word what to do and what not to do. You have also seen not so great surgeons show you what not to do. Take the good from the best of your teachers and recognize what the poorer teachers have shown you what to avoid doing. Incorporate these lessons to formulate your own surgical "rules." I have found that when I did not follow my own set of rules, trouble could ensue. Do not cut corners!

I have always felt the presence of my residency chairman looking over my shoulder to keep me from breaking the rules and committing an error.

Never Think of a Procedure as "Just" a Simple Procedure

If you start a "minor" procedure thinking it is "just" a D&C, LEEP, or whatever seems a simple procedure, you may end up turning a quick and easy case into some thing that could ruin your day as well as your patient's. Be careful and do not let your mind wander to the next thing on your schedule.

Trust Yourself: But Also Know Your Limits

Trust your knowledge and surgical experience. You have seen yourself perform skillful procedures in the past and you can do it again. There is an old saying that any obstetrician or gynecologist who denies ever perforating a uterus is either a liar or has not done very many procedures. I admit that I have had my share of perforated uteri over the years. But I have realized that almost every time that complication occurred, it was because I did not trust myself. I incorrectly convinced myself that the uterine cavity was deeper than I thought.

You will know when you are about to go past your limits. Know when to quit, ask for help, or abandon the effort to complete the surgery. There is no shame in asking for assistance before you get into trouble. That is far better than causing a complication and asking someone to correct your mistake. Do no harm!

It Is Easier to Stay Out of Trouble than to Get Out of Trouble

No explanation needed!

Take Care of Your Team

If you have not already figured this out, the people you work with can make or break you. The nurses, OR techs, anesthesia personnel, and other hospital staff are key to any of your success. Treat them right and they will reciprocate. Treat them wrong and you will regret it.

Teach the members of the team. You will have new information and new ways of accomplishing your surgical goals and the other members of the team will appreciate your desire to help them learn more.

When things do not go perfectly, keep cool! I have been asked why I did not lose my temper when problems arose with surgery. My reply was that if I thought screaming or blaming others would stop uncontrolled bleeding or make a difficult dissection easier, I would have tried that.

Avoid Disaster in the Operating Room While Training Residents

It was not that long ago that you were a new resident, looking for surgeons to allow you to operate, and now you are on the other side of that equation. How do you balance your relative inexperience as the person in charge with the opportunity to help residents gain their own experience? It can be tricky. I remember a former resident of mine coming to me after he had become an outstanding surgeon in his own right, asking me how I had had the courage to let him do any part of procedures when he was a new resident.

You have to be able to balance the resident's ability with your ability to maintain control as he or she operates. You cannot "give away" any of the surgical steps until you are confident that you can keep the resident from making any serious blunders. Not every resident will have the same degree of skills and you will have to recognize the individual's knowledge and skill level.

New Technology Is Inevitable

As you leave your training, you are probably proficient in the latest procedures and technology. Guess what? New technology is just around the corner, and you will have to figure out a way to master the new "toys" without having the safety net of being a resident. You will need a mentor who has the requisite new skill to help you until you can garner enough experience to safely go on your own.

Letting your patient know the situation is only proper, and you must assure her that her safety is paramount.

The Surgeon Is Often the Last One to Recognize That a Patient Needs to Return to the Operating Room

As we said earlier, those possible complications listed in the consent form do sometimes occur. That is how they got to be listed in the consent form. When complications do arise post operatively, swallow your pride and do whatever is necessary to remedy the problem.

Have Fun and Do Good Things

Doing good things for your patients and having fun while doing them should be your goal every day that you go to work. If you are not accomplishing these two things, try to figure out why.

Self-Evaluate Post Procedure

After every delivery or operative procedure, take a long hard look at your performance. How could you have done better? What should you have done differently? How can you correct any issues that you were not completely happy with?

If you complete a skillful, totally successful procedure, do not get too impressed with yourself. There is another case out there waiting to bite you in the butt.

If you have some difficulty in a case, analyze what you could have done differently and do not get too down on yourself. You have the knowledge and experience to improve your performance next time.

Conclusion

You can do this! Your surgical cases will not always be perfect, but following these axioms will help you to prevent disaster in the operating room. Each procedure you do will have its own obstacles and hurdles, and the experience and knowledge that you have accumulated during your training will help you to clear these hurdles.

Chapter 31
Finding the Balance of Letting Residents Operate, While Managing Patient Safety

Amanda Malik

There are many benefits to working with residents in and out of the OR. If you're reading this chapter, it's likely because you've decided to accept a role at a teaching hospital or are at least considering it. For many of us, this environment is the most familiar, as we are the recipients of such teaching during our training. As a new attending, it can be either comforting or challenging to find yourself in a new role in the same familiar hierarchy—in fact, it's likely that you will experience some element of each. This chapter attempts to offer a guide in striking the balance between letting residents operate and maintaining patient safety.

First, it is important to determine where your confidence and competence lies, as well as where it ends. It is very difficult, if not impossible, to teach or guide a resident through a case that you yourself do not know how to do. Especially as a new attending, there may be cases that either due to complexity or limited experience you do not feel ready to teach. This is ok. Of course, learning doesn't end with residency. For these cases, it is best to seek support from a partner or more experienced surgeon. Ask them to scrub with you, to do the surgery as a co-case, or even to take it on themselves but allow you to assist. For these cases, be up front with the resident team. You may want to schedule it for a time when residents are not generally available, such as during their protected education time, or let them know ahead of time that you expect they will have limited involvement. This may result in having no or very junior resident assistance, but that will allow you to focus on developing your own skills and will prevent a buildup of animosity from more senior residents.

On the contrary, if there are cases or surgeries you have a particular expertise in, then you may want to "advertise" this to the residents. You may allow them to "double" scrub with both a senior and a junior resident, or offer to cover resident clinic

A. Malik (✉)
Department of Obstetrics and Gynecology, Cooper Medical School of Rowan University and Cooper University Health Care, Camden, NJ, USA
e-mail: Malik-Amanda@cooperhealth.edu

A. Malik et al. (eds.), *An Obstetrician/Gynecologist's Path*,
https://doi.org/10.1007/978-3-031-87098-9_31

patient cases that fit your expertise. Quickly building up experience operating with residents during cases you feel most comfortable with can help you develop and strengthen your OR teaching style and confidence.

Second, get to know your residents as well as you can. This will obviously be easier in smaller programs, but luckily ob/gyn residency is 4 years—that usually allows adequate time to get to know each other. Since you will likely be at a deficit when you first start, you may want to solicit feedback from your partners or even the Program Director or Assistant Program Director. While you don't want someone else's opinion to color your own unfairly, getting information about what strengths and weaknesses various residents have shown in the OR will help you prepare for operating with them. For a resident who is known to have strong laparoscopic skills, you may hand over the camera and have them two-handed operate from the start. Conversely, for a resident who is struggling with basic surgical skills, you may have them take more of an assistant role during open cases and focus your teaching on their knot tying and suturing.

Remember that residents often learn at various paces. You cannot assume that every chief resident is highly skilled, and similarly there may be junior residents who surprise you with their surgical acumen. Some PGY-2s may outperform PGY-3s in certain cases; therefore, getting to know residents individually will help you to adapt your teaching style for each.

Third, maintain flexibility. You know by now that the course and outcome of a case is not always predictable and can sometimes surprise you. Therefore, keeping an open mind during a surgery can help you to maximize both resident experience and patient safety. For example, you may have set the expectation during an anticipated difficult case that the resident would be primarily assisting—however, if you find that it's going much smoother than anticipated, that doesn't mean you have to keep your role as primary surgeon. That may be a good opportunity to allow the resident to step up and operate. The opposite is also true. If you had anticipated an easy case but find yourself or the team to be getting into trouble, then it is of utmost importance to know when to take over. In general, if you begin to question whether what's happening is safe, then that is an appropriate time to step in. Doing so doesn't mean all educational opportunities are lost. Verbalizing your thought process can help learners to think critically and develop their own troubleshooting skills. If the urgency of the situation does not allow for that, then consider debriefing the case with the resident(s) who assisted you.

Lastly, give honest, timely, and direct feedback. Nobody benefits from being told they are "good" or "operating at expected level." If you aren't sure where to start, ask the resident what they thought went well and what they want to improve; this is a good starting point for feedback conversations and can help you assess the resident's self-awareness. If the surgery revealed a glaring deficit, spend a few minutes reviewing the bereft skill. You may demonstrate and have them practice knots, for example, or review videos of laparoscopic cases. Doing at least some feedback immediately after the case is typically most effective, as it is fresh in both of your minds. Remember that if you're at an academic institution, or even just academic-affiliated, part of your role is to train future surgeons. Therefore, it isn't just the safety of the current patient on the table at stake, but many future patients cared for by your trainees.

For many ob/gyn residents, getting to "do" a case in the OR feels like a reward for the hard work and long hours. If you're someone who enjoys the gynecology side of our field, you can probably remember the satisfaction and pride of getting to do a particularly challenging or interesting case. Try not to forget that feeling, as maintaining the memory of the role of the residents will help you in fairly determining what they do in the OR while making sure your patients receive the highest standard of care.

Chapter 32
Making Difficult Decisions in Obstetrics

Richard Fischer

Introduction

Obstetrics is one of, if not the most, challenging specialties in all of medicine. We are the only specialty that is tasked with taking care and optimizing the outcomes of two patients simultaneously, each with their own distinctive needs. This can lead to multiple clinical and ethical dilemmas, and it is often left to the OB/GYN attending to explain these difficult situations to our patients and their partners and help them to reach the decision that is right for them. Just a few of the quandaries we face include periviable deliveries and when to offer obstetrical intervention, mode of delivery for Category II/III fetal heart rate tracings, invasive versus non-invasive aneuploidy screening/testing, and of course, the religiously and politically charged issue of abortion.

One of the scariest moments after graduating a residency is when you are at the bedside of a challenging patient, you turn around, and realize you do NOT have an attending behind you to help guide your management. It can feel pretty lonely. If you make the right decision, you will be hailed as a clinical genius by your patient, and you will feel great about yourself. But if you are wrong, it will shake you to the core. Not only will you second-guess all of your decisions, but all of your decisions may be publicly second-guessed by hospital Morbidity and Mortality and/or Quality Improvement Committees, and as is too often the case within Obstetrics, by malpractice attorneys as well. It is doubtful that anyone outside of medicine can fully appreciate the loneliness that we feel in such critical moments, as well as the devastation we feel when the outcome is poor.

R. Fischer (✉)
Division of Maternal-Fetal Medicine, Department of Obstetrics and Gynecology, Cooper Medical School of Rowan University and Cooper University Health Care, Camden, NJ, USA
e-mail: fischer-richard@cooperhealth.edu

A. Malik et al. (eds.), *An Obstetrician/Gynecologist's Path*,
https://doi.org/10.1007/978-3-031-87098-9_32

The purpose of this chapter is to review the tenets of decision-making, discuss some examples of challenging clinical scenarios, and address some controversies when dealing with difficult decisions in Obstetrics.

Paternalism, Non-directed Counseling, and Shared Decision-Making

We have come a long way from the days of Marcus Welby MD (a 1970's TV series about a kindly but paternalistic physician who would make decisions for his patients). As opposed to paternalism, patient autonomy is one of the key tenets of medical ethics, whereby patients have the right to make decisions involving their bodies and their health. The next buzz word to come along was "non-directed" counseling, where physicians educated their patients about options and the patients were allowed to choose. This was a great improvement over directed counseling, but the pendulum swung too far in the direction of the physician taking no stance on the matter and allowing an individual without medical training to make a nuanced decision that might have life-altering implications. We have now moved more toward the center with "shared decision-making," where physicians and their patients work together to make a decision that is mutually agreed upon. This still requires patient education about options, while allowing physicians to make recommendations which the patient can accept or reject. It is because of this concept that I bristle at practitioners "offering" a cesarean for a Category II fetal heart rate tracing. We are not impartial restaurant servers offering something from Column A or Column B. We are highly trained professionals who know much more about fetal heart rate interpretation than our patients will ever know. Simply offering them a choice without making a recommendation is in my mind a disservice to your patients. We need to acknowledge that we do not necessarily have the one right answer, but we can explain the rationale behind our recommendations and allow the patient to make the final decision. Of course, there are some other scenarios where we cannot make recommendations, such as whether or not to terminate a pregnancy that is complicated by a fetal malformation or aneuploidy. In these cases, there is no physician expertise regarding the best course of action. Here, we can only provide our patients up-to-date information, acknowledging that we cannot predict long-term outcomes, and allow the patient to decide, with our role being to support whatever decision they make.

What Would You Do If It Was You/Your Spouse?

Don't fall into that trap! We are often asked by patients what we would do in a similar clinical circumstance. I steadfastly refuse to answer this question, though I decline it politely. I explain that we each come with our own biases and moral/

ethical backgrounds, and what is right for me might not be right for her. Additionally, I like to believe that I treat every patient the way I would for a family member. Similarly, you may be asked what others have chosen to do. Again, the answer should be the same, for every patient is unique, and what matters is whether the decision is right for the patient in front of you.

What If You Disagree with the Patient's Decision?

We strive to educate our patients so that they can be well-informed when making shared decisions. However, sometimes we might personally disagree with the patient's desires. This situation might be encountered when a prenatal patient annnounces that she would decline blood transfusion for obstetrical hemorrhage, even in life-threatening situations. While we might not make a similar choice, this is a personal patient decision that should be respected. However, if this decision makes the provider uncomfortable, they should not be forced to act in a way that deviates from her/his own moral values. In that situation, the provider should assist with transferring the patient to another practitioner who would abide by her wishes. Another hot button issue is abortion. Every person must make their own personal decision about their participation, but in those situations where it creates a moral conflict for the provider, we are obligated to assist in transferring care to an alternate provider who will honor the patient's desires.

In some cases, the patient's request might deviate from standard of care. For example, if a patient at 21 weeks with a fetus with severe early growth restriction requested a cesarean section at 21 weeks, it is unlikely that any provider would be willing to perform a cesarean at that previable gestational age. In that situation, it would be the responsibility of the provider to attempt to re-educate that patient, provide literature buttressing their position, and offer the patient the opportunity to self-transfer to another provider, as it is unlikely the provider would be able to find another practitioner who would abide with the patient's wishes.

Patient Relationships Are Key: Work as a Team

It is commonly taught that the greatest prevention of a medical malpractice suit is a good physician-patient relationship. This gets back to earlier comments about shared decision-making. This is a partnership, and if the patient feels that she has a say in her health care decisions and that you care deeply about the outcome, it can go a long way when the outcome is unfavorable.

Doing "Everything"

When dealing with a periviable gestational age, no words are as disturbing to me as "the patient wants everything done." This is a lay phrase that should be abandoned. There are so many aspects to the care of the periviable pregnancy that it is a disservice to lump them all together under "everything." When counseling a patient with periviable preterm labor or PPROM, this should be broken down into obstetrical and neonatal components. From an obstetrical perspective, would the patient want fetal monitoring, and at what gestational age would that start? If FHR monitoring is performed, would the patient wish to act on the information, including a cesarean section for a Category II/III FHR tracing? Does the patient understand the implications of a cesarean at such an early gestational age, including the potential for a Classical or even a T-incision, which would necessitate future cesareans and increase the possibility of a future uterine rupture or placenta accreta spectrum? If she desires a vaginal delivery and the fetus is in breech presentation, is she prepared for the possibility of a head entrapment, as the fetal head is typically larger than the abdomen at this early gestational age? Would she agree to a Dührssen incision, which could lead to cervical extension and future obstetrical implications? There are patients who might reasonably elect to avoid obstetrical intervention but would want neonatal resuscitation. In that scenario, it would be reasonable to offer steroids to reduce the risk of RDS, IVH, and NEC; penicillin to reduce the risk of early-onset GBS sepsis; and magnesium sulfate for neuroprotection, but no fetal monitoring until a later date. And what degree of neonatal resuscitation would she want? A neonatal consult is important to discuss anticipated survival, both with and without long-term disabilities, and to discuss interventions such as positive pressure ventilation, chest compression, and epinephrine and/or surfactant administration. The use of steroids, penicillin, or magnesium sulfate for optimization of the neonate needs to be uncoupled from the discussion of obstetrical intervention.

Just Because You Can, Doesn't Mean You Should

There is no clinical scenario more challenging than when faced with a patient who presents to OB Triage with an agonal FHR tracing. This scenario is very different from patients with a Category III tracing who are already in L&D, such as a patient with a uterine rupture or prolapsed cord, where we can get the patient back within a few minutes and in most cases deliver a vigorous infant or one that is more likely to be successfully resuscitated. A patient walking in off the street with a FHR in the 40's–50's on the monitor or one that can only be seen weakly fluttering on ultrasound can be our worst scenario. Reflexes kick in, and the tendency is to whisk the patient back for a stat cesarean. But what outcome are we anticipating, and is the patient aware of the nuances of a decision for an emergent surgery? Outcome would likely depend on the best assessment of gestational age, which can be a challenge for a patient with no prenatal care, as well as the cause for the severe prolonged deceleration/bradycardia and other maternal co-morbidities. Is there a severe abruption noted, which would likely be associated with a coagulopathy, making cesarean section more dangerous for the patient? Management of such a case is very difficult, but you must take a few moments to have a discussion with the patient about your concerns for the infant's outcome and the potential sequelae of an emergent cesarean. While many patients will reflexively request that an attempt be made to salvage the fetus, in some cases it may be advisable to recommend non-intervention, and let nature take its course. Adding to the anxiety is that we cannot know if the fetus will die as anticipated, or if it might survive and be left with long-term issues from the episode. It still behooves us to take the few moments needed to have this discussion. Given that the prolonged deceleration/bradycardia was likely present for an extended period prior to arrival in L&D, the few extra seconds of counseling will likely not make a large difference in the outcome of the infant, and will help solidify your patient's wishes.

It Is OK to Say You Don't Know and to Ask for Help

It is said that Benjamin Franklin knew everything there was to know about science and medicine, probably because there was not much known at the time. This has changed to the point that we can only know a small fraction of medicine as a whole or even within the field of Obstetrics. However, we have something that Ben did not have: the internet. The ability to search and get evidence-based answers to many of our questions has revolutionized the practice of medicine. But sometimes, in the heat of the moment, or even in an office setting, we cannot deduce the answer to a thorny clinical dilemma. This is not the time to be proud. Ask your colleagues, mentors, or experienced clinicians to weigh in on the problem. You will be more admired to be seen as someone who doesn't have all the answers, but is humble enough to ask for help.

Never Guarantee Outcomes

While we always want to give our patients hope, in the field of Obstetrics, there are no guarantees. Obstetrics is simply too unpredictable, and it is better to be uncertain than to be wrong. It is reasonable to say that you anticipate a favorable or unfavorable outcome, but don't let overconfidence lead you to promise any outcome. It is all about probabilities, not certainties.

Document, Document, Document

You have just spent a great deal of time interpreting the clinical history, examining your patient, reviewing the labs, coming up with a plan, and discussing with the patient the plan of action. Well done. Now comes the tedious part, which is documenting the entire process. As residents, you have become skilled as reporters and interpreters, but just as important is the documentation of your thought process and discussion with the patient. This is not "cover your ass" documentation, but rather documentation that allows someone else, such as a colleague, resident, or God forbid, a lawyer, to understand why you are following that course of action and the interplay between you and the patient to arrive at your shared decision-making. Though it is not as exciting as the patient interaction, it is vitally important to memorialize the discussion of risks and benefits, and may even help to crystalize your own thinking in the process. And if it helps protect you during any future litigation, that is an added bonus.

Obstetrics Is 95% Boredom and 5% Panic

This was the adage that was taught to me in medical school decades ago, and it is completely false! First of all, a good obstetrician should never be bored. As experience has likely taught you during residency, obstetrics can go from 0 to 100 mph in seconds flat. So a good practitioner should always be on her/his toes, anticipating what could go wrong at any given moment, and anticipating the actions that should be taken in the event of an emergency. Second, you should never panic. You have to be the clear-headed person in the room when all else is falling apart around you. Whether it be a severe shoulder dystocia, a ruptured uterus during a TOLAC, or a prolapsed cord, you need to think logically and sequentially of the steps that need to be taken. To quote from the classic movie Apollo 13, "Let's work the problem, people." When others see the "captain of the ship" as being calm and collected, it can only help quell the disquiet they are experiencing. Of course, you may be tightly clenching your own anal sphincter, but keep your nerves (and poop) inside.

Heavy Is the Head That Wears the Crown

There will inevitably be times when the outcome is less than ideal, resulting in either maternal or perinatal morbidity or mortality. The responsibility we all feel for our patients can lead to horrible feelings of guilt, remorse, and second-guessing. If we do not feel these emotions, we are probably not as connected to our patients as we should be. The challenge is not letting these negative emotions overcome you. People react differently to these traumas. Some outwardly express their sorrow, some bury them behind intellectual rationalizing and internalize their feelings. Unfortunately, some turn to other outlets, such as alcohol or drugs to ease their pain. Sadly, OB/GYN has one of the highest rates of physician burn-out. While there is no one answer that works for all, you should know that everyone has experienced loss in their role as a physician, whether it be directly, indirectly, or unrelated to our actions. Many institutions have services, either peer or professional, to help deal with physicians who have been traumatized by a loss. The important thing to remember is that you are not alone. And please be kind to yourself.

Conclusion

It is impossible to discuss all difficult decisions in Obstetrics, as there are so many and so varied in nature. The overriding theme in any challenging clinical dilemma is to keep a cool head, discuss the options with the patient to arrive at a shared decision for management, ask for outside help when needed, be humble enough to recognize that you will not always make the right decision, and be forgiving of yourself when the outcome is less than optimal. The bad news is that no one will ever be the master of all of Obstetrics. The good news is that you are in for one hell of a ride striving to reach that unobtainable goal. Enjoy the journey.

Chapter 33
Delivering Bad News and End-of-Life Care

David Warshal

Obstetrician/gynecologists are witness to some of the happiest moments of their patients' lives. The longitudinal nature of their care further deepens these bonds as some practitioners will care for multiple generations of a family over decades. This professional intimacy can make the always difficult job of delivering bad medical news and assisting in end-of-life decision-making even more distressing. Despite the recognition that the care provider's sensitivity and compassion play a significant role in the understanding and acceptance of bad news, there remains little formal medical training in this regard.

As a gynecologic oncologist, I frequently need to deliver bad news to my patients and assist in their end-of-life care. It is important to recognize that, for instance, recurrence of a cancer or the need to discuss end-of-life issues should not be viewed by the care provider as failure as much as the inevitable result of the disease process. When approached in this manner, the discussion becomes an opportunity to provide patients and their families with comfort, support, and guidance rather than an admission of failure on the part of the care provider. As I frequently tell my residents and fellows, success in oncology is often not about whether the patient has been cured but is always about the compassion, respect, and skill underlying each encounter.

The patient-centered decision-making model with the patient involved in all aspects of their management represents the standard of care in the United States since the latter half of the twentieth century. Patient surveys since then have almost uniformly revealed patients' strong desire for information regarding their diagnosis and prognosis. However, personal and/or cultural differences often dictate the extent

D. Warshal (✉)
Division of Gynecologic Oncology, MD Anderson Cancer Center at Cooper, Cooper Medical School of Rowan University and Cooper University Health Care, Camden, NJ, USA

A. Malik et al. (eds.), *An Obstetrician/Gynecologist's Path*,
https://doi.org/10.1007/978-3-031-87098-9_33

of information a patient desires and whether they would like family members to participate in discussions and decision-making.

There are a variety of protocols developed to assist clinicians in delivering bad news. With each, it is important that the caregiver engages the patient in a compassionate, supportive manner while providing accurate information. Studies indicate that frank conversations managed properly can result in longer survival with an improved quality of life.

The SPIKES protocol was developed in part at the MD Anderson Cancer Center as a six-step protocol for delivering bad news to cancer patients. For maximum benefit, the plan is dependent upon completion of each step before progressing to the next step. The methodology is equally applicable to other discussions within the OB/Gyn realm such as pregnancy loss and infertility.

Step 1: Setting Up the Meeting

When preparing to give bad news, it is ideal to arrange for an in-person meeting while avoiding significant delays in delivering this information. The patient should be asked beforehand if they would like family or friends to be present. Meetings should be in a quiet, private setting to avoid interruptions with adequate time scheduled to allow for questions. If the meeting follows an examination, the patient should be allowed to dress prior to starting the conversation. Patients lacking decision-making capacity should have their legal decision-maker with them. Other practitioners directly involved in relevant aspects of the patient's management, such as a palliative care provider, should be invited. The leader of the meeting is usually the individual who is most familiar with the patient and their medical condition, able to answer questions regarding risks and benefits of management options and discuss prognosis. The leader and any other caregivers involved in the discussion should sit at the same level or lower than the patient and maintain eye contact when speaking. When appropriate, touching an arm or holding a hand can be very effective as well.

Step 2: Perception

At the start, the clinician aims to gain information about the patient's understanding of their condition. Use open-ended questions with gentle probing to identify misperceptions, unrealistic expectations, or denial that, if necessary, can be addressed later in the meeting. An example is asking "What is your understanding of your medical condition?"

Step 3: Invitation

Patients vary in their desire to receive information regarding their medical condition. Ask for permission from the patient to provide information (i.e., May I give you the test results?) and allow the patient to communicate the extent of detail that they desire (i.e., Would you like all the details or just a summary and focus on my plan?). Providing information to family members or other trusted confidants at the patient's request can also be extremely helpful.

Step 4: Knowledge

I find it beneficial to summarize the events leading up to the meeting. It ensures that everyone in the meeting understands the issues and allows me to address any misperceptions identified in step two. I also take this opportunity to further educate the patient regarding their disease, provide positive reinforcement, and give a warning that bad news is coming. An example would be a statement such as the following: "As we have discussed, ovarian cancer is very difficult to treat. Despite doing everything we have recommended, your recent CT results are not what we hoped for."

It is particularly important to refrain from using technical jargon and to adjust the level of conversation to that of the patient's understanding. Providing information gently and in limited amounts at a time aids in patients' understanding and retention. It is often helpful to confirm with the patient that they understand. In addition, it is important to maintain an appropriately positive attitude and offer management options that may benefit the patient. For individuals for whom no additional therapy is indicated, discussing pain management, symptom relief, and hospice may provide great comfort.

Step 5: Emotions

Patients are encouraged to express their emotions with appropriate empathetic and validating responses from their caregiver. The emotions can include shock, anger, and grief. I find that if there has been effective communication with the patient throughout their treatment and if the earlier steps were well managed, the primary emotion experienced by the patient and their family is sadness in the acknowledgment of their condition. I will often let them know how sorry I am to have to break such unfortunate news while validating their emotions with a supportive response.

Step 6: Strategy and Summary

A summary of the prior five steps is an opportunity for patients and their families to refocus and allows the clinician to address any persistent misperceptions. In this age of shared decision-making, it is important to realistically address prognosis as this may have a significant impact on strategy moving forward. This discussion can be very difficult, particularly when viable treatment options are not available or when the patient's performance status does not allow ongoing treatment. Under such dire circumstances, it is important to recognize that you as the caregiver have a critical role in helping patients and their family make important end-of-life decisions. I have found that the kindness and compassion expressed in these situations is always especially appreciated by patients and families.

As patients transition from active therapeutic management to purely palliative care, end-of-life decision-making becomes the primary focus. However, under ideal circumstances, planning for catastrophic medical illness and death should have begun much earlier. As outlined by the National Institute on Aging's checklist for getting your affairs in order, advanced planning prior to an illness includes steps such as (1) estate planning with drafting a will and designating a durable power of attorney for finances; (2) preparing a living will and choosing a healthcare proxy; (3) discussing advance care planning with your healthcare providers; (4) providing a trusted caregiver with permission to speak with your caregivers, lawyer, and various financial institutions; and (5) placing all important papers and legal documents in a single secure location. These steps will help to ensure that the individual's healthcare and financial interests are managed in a manner commensurate with their desires. They will also relieve the burden that often falls on family members when their loved one becomes incapacitated, and these steps have not been taken.

Over the past 50 years, much has changed in how we view death and dying. In 1967, the first hospice was established in the United Kingdom, where the hospice movement had begun. Dr. Elizabeth Kubler-Ross published her groundbreaking book *On Death and Dying*, which identifies the five stages through which many terminally ill patients progress—denial, anger, bargaining, depression, and acceptance—in 1969. The first hospice was established in the United States in 1974, but it was not until 1982 that the US Congress passed a provision to create a Medicare hospice benefit. This was made permanent 3 years later. It was during this time and beyond that legal decisions involving Karen Ann Quinlan, Nancy Cruzan, and others established the case law that allows for self-determination by either the individual or by their healthcare proxy in the matter of continuing or withdrawing life sustaining treatments. Though it remains controversial, Oregon in 1994 was the first of several states to enact legislation that allows physicians to assist in the death of mentally capable, terminally ill patients by providing the means and/or information to enable the patient to perform the life-ending act. Opposed to medical aid in dying for many years, the American Medical Association (AMA) issued a new policy position in June 2019 affirming that physicians can medically aid in dying "according to the dictates of their conscience without violating their professional obligations."

Within this context, there has been significant medical and lay interest in what has been termed a "good death." Though there are multiple definitions, the Institute of Medicine defines a good death as "one that is free from avoidable distress and suffering, for patients, family and caregivers; in general accord with the patients' and families' wishes; and reasonably consistent with clinical, cultural and ethical standards."

A model to promote a good death was proposed in 1998 by Emanuel and Emanuel. It identified fixed patient characteristics, modifiable dimensions of the patient's experience and care system interventions that can be used to support a dying patient (Fig. 33.1).

Many subsequent studies have examined patients' perspectives on core elements of a good death and compared them to those of family members and caregivers. Pain and symptom management, clear decision-making, autonomy, a feeling of closure, and preparation for death were important to all groups in most studies. The importance assigned to issues such as spirituality, dying at home, and maintaining mental awareness varied among the groups. Of interest, patients were more concerned about maintaining mental awareness than their caregivers with the opposite being true for dying at home.

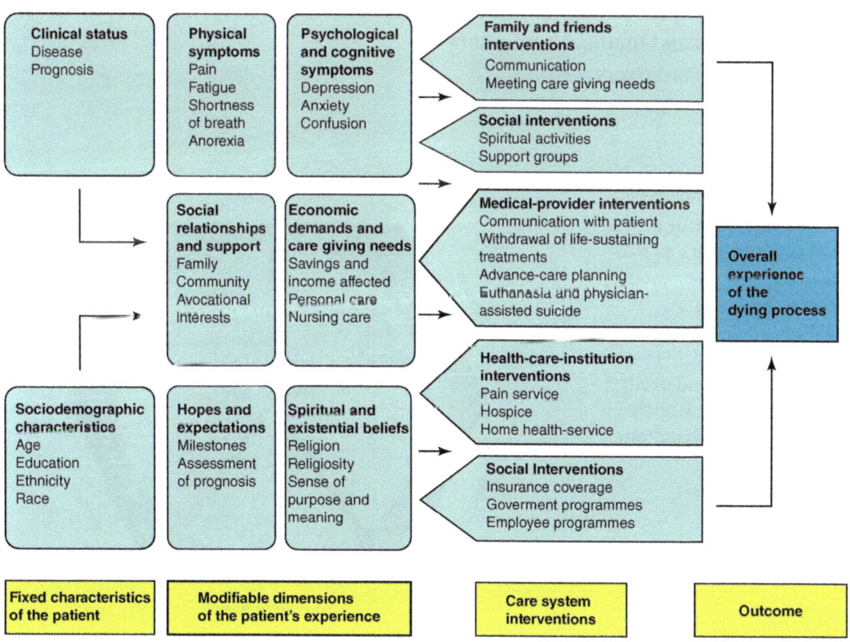

Fig. 33.1 Framework for a good death. (Source: Emanuel EJ, Emanuel LJ. The promise of a good death. Lancet. 1998;351:SII21–SII29)

A 2020 review of the literature identified five core elements that were common to most patients' notion of a good death and five secondary factors that influenced the core elements. Researchers found that the secondary factors of culture, religion, age, life circumstances, disease, and finances strongly affected the importance placed on the associated core element. As an example, the authors pointed out that concern for control of pain and other symptoms was of great significance to individuals with limited access to healthcare but of much less concern to those with well-established medical care. They concluded that the most important aspects to a good death were highly individualized based on a variety of personal and cultural circumstances and varied for the individual based upon where they were in the dying process (Fig. 33.2).

Hospice care is now generally considered the quality end-of-life healthcare option. It provides expert medical care, symptom management, and emotional and spiritual support that is individualized to the needs and desires of the patient and their family. Patients become eligible if they agree to supportive care only and their life expectancy is 6 months or less. Services are available regardless of illness or demographics. A family member or close associate serves as the primary caregiver and is supported by the hospice staff and volunteers who regularly visit to assess the patient's needs. A care plan is initiated by the hospice physician or medical director with support from an interdisciplinary team (Fig. 33.3).

Services include the following:

- Pain and symptom management
- Emotional, psychosocial, and spiritual support for the patient and their loved ones
- Medications and medical equipment
- Training of caregivers

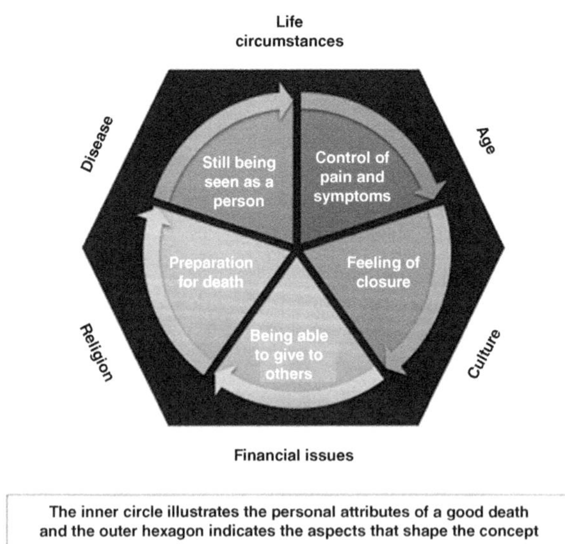

Fig. 33.2 Categories of analysis (core elements or personal attributes of a good death and factors that shape the concept). (Source: Krikorian A, Maldonado C, Pastrana T. Patient's perspectives on the notion of a good death: a systematic review of the literature. J Pain Symptom Manage. 2020;59(1):152–64)

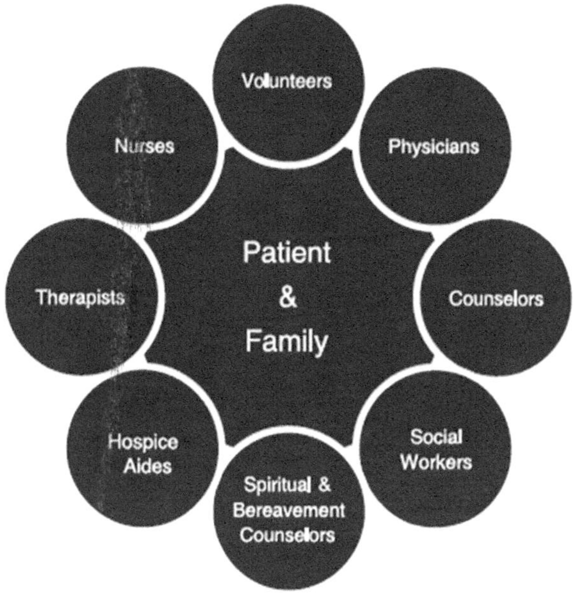

Fig. 33.3 Structure of the interdisciplinary team

- Grief support and counseling of family and friends for up to 13 months following death
- Provide residential care that can be escalated to continuous home care for between 8 and 24 hours a day to manage acute symptoms, respite care with brief admissions to a care facility to provide relief to the patient's primary caregiver, and general inpatient care for management of symptoms that require more intensive care
- Provide specialized services as needed

Acceptance of hospice care in the United States has steadily increased over time. In 2021, of the over 2.7 million Medicare decedents, 52.5% of females and 42.1% of males were enrolled in hospice. White Medicare decedents used hospice in 50% of cases, while utilization among all other races ranged from 34% to 36%. Urban decedents were more likely to enroll in hospice followed by those residing in metropolitan and rural areas.

Chapter 34
Professionalism

Michelle Iavicoli

Introduction

Professionalism in the medical field may be incorporated into the residency curriculum, but it is a skill best acquired through experience, observation, and maturity. It is easy to teach a learner the practice of medicine; it takes finesse to teach the art of professionalism. Webster's dictionary defines professionalism as "the skill, good judgment and polite behavior that is expected from a person who is trained to do a job well" [1]. In this chapter, I would like to expound upon this definition by illustrating what I deem to be the foundation of professionalism in the medical profession. We begin with Experience.

Experience

Clinical Competence

As a new provider, you graduate with clinical experience taught to you by your mentors. It is now your responsibility to commit yourself to being a lifelong learner. It is up to you to maintain clinical competence over the course of your career in medicine. Practical ways to ensure maintenance and growth of clinical competence include faculty development, CME, conferences, and journal reading. Being open

M. Iavicoli (✉)
Department of Obstetrics and Gynecology, Cooper Medical School of Rowan University and Cooper University Health Care, Camden, NJ, USA
e-mail: iavicoli-michelle@cooperhealth.edu

A. Malik et al. (eds.), *An Obstetrician/Gynecologist's Path*,
https://doi.org/10.1007/978-3-031-87098-9_34

to trying new techniques is a necessary component of your competence and growth. Only you are responsible for your expertise in the practice of obstetrics and gynecology. It is now your goal to commit to ongoing lifelong professional development. As you continue to grow your medical knowledge base, so too will you grow in professionalism. Learn and grow from your accomplishments and your mistakes. Observe your mentors and mimic their professionalism, learn from their mistakes. When you see yourself well respected in your field, reflect on the qualities that you emulate and foster them, suppress those that held you back. This will make you continue to grow and be respected as a true professional.

Cultural Competence

Cultural competence is an imperative quality of a true professional. As residents, we are taught to be sensitive and respond to a patient's culture, age, and disabilities. This pursuit to understand patients and how they view the healthcare system is ongoing. Being culturally competent improves the healthcare that you provide to your patients and helps to reduce healthcare disparities. Cultural competence is often accomplished at the micro level, by seeking to understand each patient as an individual. This necessitates an awareness of medical trends in certain cultures and ethnicities. This can be as simple as knowing that thalassemia is more prevalent in the Mediterranean population, and as complex as learning about how religion impacts how a patient seeks and receives healthcare. A Jehovah's Witness religiously does not believe that blood that leaves the body should ever return to the body, hence their refusal of blood products. It is a religious belief. It is not a statement on their disbelief in medical care. Literacy and economic structure play a role in a patient's perception and acceptance of healthcare. Sometimes a simple explanation is worth more than a technical recital. Remember to always embody this awareness into your practice. A true professional will always prioritize maintenance of cultural competence. As your cultural competence grows so should your ethical competence.

Ethical Competence

Residents are also charged with demonstrating a commitment to ethical practice. What does this mean? Ethical care is care provided to your patients always in their best interest, without bias, while always being truthful and confidential. Our Hippocratic Oath states Primum Non Noncere, or "First do no harm" [2]. Never withhold clinical care, but it is your obligation to respect the values and wishes of your patient. This seems simple enough in theory but can become complicated in practice. Consider a laboring patient who refuses an operative delivery. A pregnant patient who insists on a primary cesarean section. A gynecologic patient who insists on a hysterectomy. It is our responsibility to present an unbiased approach to the pros, cons, and alternative treatments that are reasonable for each medical scenario. When the patient makes their decision, it must be honored to the best of your ability. In the event you are unable to fulfill your obligation, you owe a duty to take the necessary steps to refer the patient to a provider that can justly honor this request. This principle of patient autonomy must take precedence. You are charged with educating and empowering your patients to make appropriate medical decisions. If after you provide a balance of counseling you don't agree with the patient, suggest another professional's opinion. Remember your opinion is not always another's. Social justice plays a role as well. It is important to consider the available resources and needs of your patient while taking care of them. By committing to the practice of patient autonomy and social justice, you will commit to a career of practicing ethical medicine and will forever embody respect from your patients and peers.

Observation

Compassion and Empathy

Compassion and empathy are essential qualities of a true professional. The Co-CEOs of Cooper University Health system have succeeded in scientifically proving the value that compassion and empathy play in the success of patient care and the overall fulfillment by those providing that care. They suggest in their book titled, *Compassionomics: The Revolutionary Scientific Evidence That Caring Makes a Difference* [3], that compassion is the wonder drug of the twenty-first century. As obstetricians, we treat a vulnerable, emotionally labile group of patients. The hormonal teenager with acne. A 36-week pregnant mother of three who has back pain and is sleep deprived. The 80-year-old woman who is frustrated by the aging process. It is our responsibility to hear and relate to these concerns as physicians. I remind our residents that the five am baby may be humdrum to them, but it is a pinnacle event for that mother. Celebrate it! Embodying this emotional response in everyday practice will not only foster a stronger connection with your patients, but it will provide sustained fulfillment in your career.

Honesty and Integrity

It is our role as obstetrician gynecologists to provide care to the best of our ability while embodying honesty and integrity. In fact, integrity means our actions are honest and trustworthy. It is expected that you as a professional use judgment or expertise to always act in a responsible, reliable manner. The only way you will build trust with your patients is to always be honest and reliable. It is this integrity that will build trust throughout your career. Observe your more senior peers. How do they build trust? By embodying honesty and integrity in their everyday practices. For example, if a patient asks you for treatment options, you may feel strongly about one option, but it is your responsibility to present all reasonable options without bias. When they make their decision, accept it, and don't try to sway them your way. It is imperative that you be truthful when a mistake is made. Patients are informed that mistakes can happen. Be truthful and be honest. Patients embrace the truth and will be less apt to follow a litigious path. A professional career built on honesty and integrity will flourish for decades to come.

Maturity

Accountability

We learn professionalism as we mature. Maturity breeds accountability. As physicians, we are trained to take responsibility for those for whom we provide care. Listen to your patients more than you speak. Give them their time to tell their stories. Take detailed notes, don't cut them off, and accept what they have to say. Follow up with them in a timely manner. Respond to their questions with meaning and interest rather than complacency and annoyance. But accountability does not only apply to your relationship with your patients but with yourself. Be accountable for you and your actions. Respond positively to feedback, embrace change, and admit your mistakes. Be aware that poor communication with your patients and peers lacks accountability and in turn professionalism. Fostering hazing and hierarchical practice with your peers proves you to have no personal accountability. If you value your personal accountability, you foster respect from your patients, collaborate better with your peers, and uphold the true core of professionalism.

Punctuality

If early is on time, then on time is late. As a provider, you will invariably be busy. But remember, your patients and colleagues are equally as busy as you are. See your patients on time. Arrive at your meetings five minutes early. Sign in for the operating room with ample time for your patients to ask questions, your staff to confirm your supplies, and your residents to review the procedure. This practice will not only gain the respect of your patients, but command respect from your staff and peers. In turn, they will return the respect with timely arrival to your office, efficiency in the operating room, and support in the office. A true professional sees the value of other's time equivalent to their time.

Demeanor

Did the surgeon who yells in the operating room gain or lose your confidence in his skills? Most likely lose. Be calm. Even under times of stress. Adrenaline will get the best of all of us, but don't let it consume you. In times of stress, take a breath, think clearly, and proceed. Chances are you will manage any crisis in a safer, collaborative way. No one gets things done by yelling and screaming. It will turn your team on you. Rather, a calm demeanor will exude control and professionalism, which is always a win in the end.

Conclusion

In summary, professionalism is not a learned trait, but an acquired one. Always look for the opportunity to be a professional. Use your experience, observation, and maturity to grow your clinical acumen, compassion, empathy, and honesty. Try to remain accountable for yourself and others. Your demeanor will capture the true you as a professional. Remain calm and in command, and you too will be the true professional.

Good Luck!

References

1. Merriam-Webster. Professionalism. In: Merriam-Webster.com dictionary. 2024. Retrieved 12 Feb 2024, from https://www.merriam-webster.com/dictionary/professionalism.
2. Oxford Reference. Primum non nocere. Retrieved 13 Feb 2024, from https://www.oxfordreference.com/view/10.1093/oi/authority.20110803100345841.
3. Trzeciak S, Mazzarelli A, Booker C. Compassionomics: the revolutionary scientific evidence that caring makes a difference. Huron Consulting Services LLC; 2019.

Chapter 35
A Guide for Being Minorities in Medicine: Advancing Diversity, Equity, and Inclusion for Ourselves and Our Patients

Karissa Rajagopal, Kyle Le, Tyler Cholankeril, and Guy Hewlett

Background

Diversity, Equity, and Inclusion (DEI) have been recent considerations in obstetrics and gynecology (Ob-Gyn) as with all medical specialties. In the United States (U.S.), Ob-Gyn residency training became a requirement for independent practice by the middle of the twentieth century, and several decades thereafter, residency training programs were white and male dominated [1]. Women, minority groups, and openly lesbian, gay, bisexual, transgender, queer/questioning, intersex, asexual, and other (LGBTQIA+) individuals faced a myriad of barriers to entry and advancement into residency for all medical specialties. There were also barriers for these groups for admission into medical school.

A confluence of social events and legal policies drove broad-scale change in many sectors during the latter half of the twentieth century. The civil rights movement of the late 1950s and 1960s brought an unprecedented focus on issues of discrimination and inequality in many sectors including healthcare [2]. This new attention forced many institutions to reassess their approach to screening, recruitment, and admissions in response to changing societal attitudes and pressure to promote inclusivity. Affirmative action policies of the 1960s and 1970s attempted to address decades of systemic discrimination and inequities against marginalized

K. Rajagopal (✉) · T. Cholankeril · G. Hewlett
Department of Obstetrics and Gynecology, Cooper Medical School of Rowan University and Cooper University Health Care, Camden, NJ, USA

K. Le
Reproductive Endocrinology and Infertility, Jones Institute at Old Dominion University, Norfolk, VA, USA

Department of Obstetrics and Gynecology, Cooper Medical School of Rowan University and Cooper University Health Care, Camden, NJ, USA

A. Malik et al. (eds.), *An Obstetrician/Gynecologist's Path*,
https://doi.org/10.1007/978-3-031-87098-9_35

groups to promote diversity in education and employment settings. Passage of the Civil Rights Act of 1964 and subsequent congressional expansion created a legal framework which prohibited discrimination based on gender, race, and other characteristics in education and employment. Advocacy groups and professional organizations played a crucial role in advancing DEI in the field of Ob-Gyn. The American College of Obstetricians and Gynecologists (ACOG) advocated for policies that promote diversity and inclusion in Ob-Gyn residency training programs.

These developments have resulted in a more diverse pool of Ob-Gyn residency applicants, and consequently, greater diversity in residency programs. Despite these advances in Ob-Gyn resident diversity, individuals from traditionally marginalized backgrounds continue to face barriers to entry and disproportionate challenges navigating residency and postgraduate careers.

Introduction

We, the authors of this chapter, are a first-generation, Indian, queer, cis-gendered female; a first-generation Vietnamese, queer, cis-gendered male; an American-born straight White female; and an Afro-Caribbean straight Black male. We have all experienced being "othered" throughout our medical careers. At times, we experienced this sense of otherness before understanding what it meant or having a vocabulary to name it. This term refers to treating someone as fundamentally different from the mainstream group [3]. In medicine, the mainstream typically comprises American-born, white, heterosexual, able-bodied, cis-gendered males. As with all people, there exist subtleties within each of our identities, and learning to recognize and appreciate these unique characteristics can simultaneously empower and uplift traditionally marginalized individuals and create a more positive work environment. The following provides a framework of important domains for building a more inclusive and supportive workspace with specific behavioral recommendations.

Minority Tax

Minority tax refers to the additional time or workload imposed on physicians from non-dominant backgrounds compared to their counterparts in the dominant group [4]. Below are examples we have experienced or witnessed, though this list is not exhaustive:

- Asking a Black person to serve on DEI committee solely due to their race.
- Asking a Spanish-speaking colleague to translate.
- Muslim professors being approached by Muslim students for mentorship, as they may feel safer with someone from a similar background.
- The only queer provider in an office being tasked with addressing all questions about LGBTQIA+ care.

For many providers, the challenge lies in the intersection between wanting to help patients or students from similar backgrounds and the desire to improve the current environment. While fulfilling in many ways, this additional "ask" may take away time from personal growth in research, patient care, and well-being [5]. This dichotomy further perpetuates the cycle of guilt and desire to "prove worth" among the dominant culture, especially in a subset already beset by imposter syndrome issues.

Physicians from non-dominant backgrounds should carefully determine the amount of time they can dedicate to volunteer activities and establish clear boundaries by becoming comfortable with declining additional commitments. If your institution is open to the idea, consider negotiating for designated time specifically allocated for these pursuits, ensuring minimal interference with your clinical responsibilities. Some institutions may consider paid compensation for DEI work.

Microaggressions

The term "microaggressions" refers to commonplace behavioral indignities that may be intentional or unintentional [6]. It is important to acknowledge the critique of the term "microaggression." The use of "micro" undervalues the gravity of the offense. Recent studies show that regular daily exposure to perceived discrimination is equal to or worse than overt discrimination. Microaggression contributes to lower self-esteem, workplace burnout, anxiety, and depression [7]. All of this to say, while the term uses micro, it does not imply small harm.

At times, it may be hard to identify when microaggressions occur. They may be brief exchanges in passing or framed as innocent curious questions. For example, "Where are you from…no, where are you really from?" "I want to see the oriental doctor," "Are you the nurse?"

The recipient, attempting to rectify the stress, may ask themselves:

- Did this person intend to insult me?
- Should I respond?
- How should I respond?
- What would happen if I say something?
- Is it worth the trouble?
- Am I making a big deal about nothing?

Dealing with this involves weighing personal safety, the other person's openness to dialogue, and the potential regret of staying silent. Often, frustration is suppressed and spilled into other aspects of work and life. Practicing tools to recognize, respond, and cope can improve outcomes for self and the culture of the institution. Torres et al. introduced a framework for recognizing and responding to microaggressions in medicine and surgery [7].

ACTION

- Ask clarifying questions.
- Come from curiosity, not judgment.
- Tell what you observed in a factual manner.
- Impact exploration—discuss what the impact of the statement was.
- Own your own thoughts and feelings around the situation.
- Share with a friend.

Mistreatment from Patients

Approximately 60% of doctors indicate that they have encountered biased comments from patients, with almost 50% noting instances where patients sought a different healthcare provider based on a specific demographic characteristic of the physician [8]. Some comments from patients are overt, including derogatory language, slurs, aggressive behavior/tone, and sexual inappropriateness. Others are subtler, such as microaggressions and "problematic compliments."

Unfortunately, these forms of assault are often left unaddressed due to various reasons, including a lack of time, uncertainty about how to intervene effectively, fear of damaging the therapeutic alliance, concern about escalating the situation, and apprehension that intervention may not receive institutional support. Additionally, there is a fear that addressing such issues could negatively impact personal or institutional metrics like Press-Ganey scores [9].

Addressing biased comments from patients requires careful consideration, as there is no one-size-fits-all approach. Personal safety and comfort should always be the top priority for healthcare providers. It is crucial to acknowledge these situations and develop strategies to address them effectively. Here are some considerations:

1. *Maintain Professionalism*
   - Always prioritize your safety and comfort.
   - Respond calmly and professionally, avoiding escalation of the situation.
   - Attempt to redirect the conversation back to the medical topic at hand.
2. *Educate and Advocate*
   - Use the incident as a teaching moment to educate patients on appropriate behavior in the healthcare setting.
   - Advocate for respect and tolerance, emphasizing the importance of a positive doctor-patient relationship.
3. *Seek Support from Colleagues*
   - Talk to department chairs, mentors, or colleagues about your experience.
   - Share your concerns and seek guidance on how to handle similar situations in the future.

4. *Establish Boundaries*
   - Clearly communicate and set boundaries for acceptable behavior during appointments.
   - If a patient crosses these boundaries, address the issue professionally and firmly.
5. *Document Incidents*
   - Keep records of any incidents, including dates, times, and details of the encounter.
   - This documentation can be useful if you need to involve higher-ups or discuss the situation with hospital administration.
6. *Report to Superiors*
   - If the situation persists or becomes severe, report the incidents to your superiors or the appropriate authorities within your healthcare institution.
   - Ensure that your institution has a process in place for addressing such concerns.
7. *Institutional Support*
   - Advocate for a supportive institutional culture that prioritizes the well-being of healthcare providers.
   - Encourage policies that address patient behavior that goes against the principles of respect and inclusivity.
8. *Legal Considerations*
   - Be aware of any legal protections in place for healthcare professionals facing discrimination.
   - Consult legal resources if the situation warrants further action.

It is important to remember that every situation is unique, and the response may vary based on the specific circumstances. The ultimate goal is to create a safe and respectful environment for both healthcare providers and patients.

Mentorship

Mentorship plays a pivotal role in facilitating career advancement, offering research guidance, and providing essential support. However, research has found that faculty from underrepresented backgrounds in medicine receive less mentoring compared to their nonminority counterparts [10]. This is supported by the 2010 AAMC report which showed lower promotion rates among nonwhite faculty members [11]. Senior faculty predominantly comprise individuals from the dominant group, resulting in a disproportionate burden on diverse faculty members to serve on numerous academic committees, task forces, and workgroups aimed at enhancing institutional diversity (referred to as the minority tax previously discussed).

Systematic reviews have evaluated best practices in mentoring modalities such as one-on-one mentorship by seasoned investigators, participation in group-based skill-building seminars, facilitation of access to pilot grants, and provision of support for conducting pilot studies. Implementing such options necessitates acknowledgment from leadership to afford protected or compensated time. Failing to address the specific mentorship needs of the non-dominant workforce further exacerbates the gap in available mentorship opportunities and networks, contributing to attrition rates among minority faculty [12]. In some cases, seeking mentorship from external organizations, such as national identity-based groups or clubs, may be necessary to supplement institutional support.

Medical Students

Underrepresented in Medicine/Black, Indigenous, and Other People of Color (URM/BIPOC) medical students disproportionately experience physical, mental, and emotional trauma as well as significantly higher rates of discrimination compared to their colleagues [13]. URM/BIPOC medical students also tend to receive lower clinical scores compared to their cohort during clerkship years [14]. These grades are subjective and are based on physicians' impressions of the student, which can be affected by implicit bias. In addition, medical students in sexual minority groups report fear of discrimination and increased mistreatment. As an attending, it is critical to be mindful of the disparities that exist within medical education and the systematic forms of oppression medical students face. Attendings can act as role models and provide mentorship to empower students. While there is inherently a power dynamic between attendings and students, there is still room for solidarity and support. In teaching settings, attendings can exhibit behaviors that create a supportive, respectful, and non-judgmental environment in which all learners feel acknowledged and validated. Furthermore, attendings can partner with student advocacy groups to help support initiatives and enhance messages of inclusion. Physicians can use their voice to help advocate for students when they may fear retribution.

What Is My Role as a White Person in DEI Initiatives?

The role of white people or any member of the dominant group in DEI initiatives is multifaceted and crucial for creating meaningful change. Here are some key aspects:

- *Recognize Privilege*: Acknowledging one's privilege and understanding how it impacts perceptions, opportunities, and experiences is essential. This recognition forms the basis of empathizing with others who may not have the same privileges. For example, in a meeting, a white male's voice may carry more weight than a female's. Similarly, a person from multiple generations of physicians may have more networking opportunities for career advancement compared to someone who is a first-generation college or medical student.

- *Allyship*: White individuals can act as allies by actively supporting marginalized communities, advocating for their rights, and amplifying their voices. This can include speaking out against discrimination, challenging biased attitudes and behaviors, and actively working to dismantle systemic barriers. One must also recognize the differences between "white savior" and true allyship—offering support rather than assuming someone wants support.
- *Education and Awareness*: This includes understanding the historical and systemic factors that contribute to inequality, as well as staying informed about current events and initiatives aimed at promoting diversity and inclusion and advocating for this education as part of a standard medical curriculum.
- *Creating Inclusive Spaces*: This involves actively promoting diversity, fostering a culture of belonging, and ensuring that everyone feels valued and respected, for example, adding various religious holidays to shared calendars, celebrating identity months (e.g., pride month and black history month). Those that sit on interview committees can advocate for training to conduct non-racist interviews and support hiring more diverse candidates.
- *Supporting Structural Change*: Addressing systemic inequities requires advocating for policy changes and institutional reforms that promote fairness and equality for all individuals, regardless of race or ethnicity. When carrying out policy changes, it is important to have people of the background you are advocating for be part of the conversation.

Patient Outcomes

We would be remiss to overlook the appalling disparate patient outcomes in a chapter on DEI in Ob-Gyn. According to the Centers for Disease Control (CDC), a Black/African-American patient is approximately three times more likely to die from complications of pregnancy, childbirth, and the postpartum period than their white counterparts. Shockingly, this disparity is even greater in some parts of the U.S., including New Jersey. Although it is difficult to ascribe these disparate outcomes to a specific cause, it is likely that there is a complex conglomeration of contributory factors including unconscious bias, lack of cultural competence, systemic racism, and disparities in access to and delivery of care. While an in-depth exploration of this inequality is beyond the scope of this chapter, it is imperative that all Ob-Gyn practitioners acknowledge this reality and adopt an attitude of humility and willingness to embrace practice improvement methodologies to dismantle the systemic barriers that have allowed this discrepancy to persist for far too long.

Conclusion

In conclusion, the imperative for Diversity, Equity, and Inclusion (DEI) initiatives in obstetrics and gynecology (Ob-Gyn) underscores the pressing need to confront entrenched disparities in healthcare. This chapter offers a historical backdrop and serves as a roadmap for providers, particularly those from historically marginalized groups, to navigate a system inherently biased against them. By shedding light on the concept of "otherness," examining the burdens of minority tax, addressing microaggressions, tackling patient mistreatment, advocating for equitable mentorship opportunities, and supporting underrepresented medical students, this chapter aims to empower physicians to challenge systemic injustices. Moreover, it emphasizes the critical role of individuals from dominant groups, such as white individuals, in driving meaningful change by recognizing privilege, practicing genuine allyship, fostering education and awareness, creating inclusive environments, and advocating for structural reforms. Through collective effort and unwavering commitment, we can strive toward a healthcare system that truly embodies the principles of diversity, equity, and inclusion for all.

References

1. Chervenak FA, Asfaw TS, Shaktman BD, McCullough LB. Gender diversity in residency training: the case for affirmative inclusion. J Grad Med Educ. 2017;9(6):685–7. https://doi.org/10.4300/JGME-D-17-00140.1. PMID: 29270254; PMCID: PMC5734319
2. Hahn RA, Truman BI, Williams DR. Civil rights as determinants of public health and racial and ethnic health equity: health care, education, employment, and housing in the United States. SSM Popul Health. 2018;4:17–24. https://doi.org/10.1016/j.ssmph.2017.10.006. PMID: 29250579; PMCID: PMC5730086
3. Talbott JMV, Wasson MN. Sex and racial/ethnic diversity in accredited obstetrics and gynecology specialty and subspecialty training in the United States. J Surg Educ. 2022;79(3):818–27. https://doi.org/10.1016/j.jsurg.2021.12.011. Accessed 12 June 2022
4. Rodríguez JE, Campbell KM, Pololi LH. Addressing disparities in academic medicine: what of the minority tax? BMC Med Educ. 2015;15:6. https://doi.org/10.1186/s12909-015-0290-9.
5. Williamson T, et al. Minority tax reform — avoiding overtaxing minorities when we need them most. N Engl J Med. 2021;384(20):1877–9. https://doi.org/10.1056/nejmp2100179. Accessed 4 Sept 2021
6. Torres MB, et al. Recognizing and reacting to microaggressions in medicine and surgery. JAMA Surg. 2019;154(9):868. jamanetwork.com/journals/jamasurgery/fullarticle/2738043, https://doi.org/10.1001/jamasurg.2019.1648
7. Ehie O, Muse I, Hill L, Bastien A. Professionalism: microaggression in the healthcare setting. Curr Opin Anaesthesiol. 2021;34(2):131–6. https://doi.org/10.1097/ACO.0000000000000966. PMID: 33630771; PMCID: PMC7984763
8. Watson S. Credentials don't shield doctors, nurses from bias. WebMD website. https://www.webmd.com/a-to-z-guides/news/20171018/survey-patient-bias-toward-doctors-nurses. Published 18 Oct 2017. Accessed 12 Feb 2019.
9. DeLoughery EP. Physician race and specialty influence Press Ganey survey results. Neth J Med. 2019;77(10):366–9. PMID: 31880269

10. Nunez-Smith M, Ciarleglio MM, Sandoval-Schaefer T, Elumn J, Castillo-Page L, Peduzzi P, Bradley EH. Institutional variation in the promotion of racial/ethnic minority faculty at US medical schools. Am J Public Health. 2012;102(5):852–8. https://doi.org/10.2105/AJPH.2011.300552. Epub 2012 Mar 15. PMID: 22420820; PMCID: PMC3483910
11. Xierali I, et al. Faculty Diversity in U.S. Medical Schools: Progress and Gaps Coexist. Dec 2016. www.aamc.org/media/8406/download
12. Bonifacino E, Ufomata EO, Farkas AH, Turner R, Corbelli JA. Mentorship of underrepresented physicians and trainees in academic medicine: a systematic review. J Gen Intern Med. 2021;36(4):1023–34. https://doi.org/10.1007/s11606-020-06478-7. Epub 2021 Feb 2. PMID: 33532959; PMCID: PMC7852467
13. O'Marr JM, Chan SM, Crawford L, Wong AH, Samuels E, Boatright D. Perceptions on Burnout and the Medical School learning environment of medical students who are underrepresented in medicine. JAMA Netw Open. 2022;5(2):e220115. https://doi.org/10.1001/jamanetworkopen.2022.0115. PMID: 35195698; PMCID: PMC8867243
14. Low D, Pollack SW, Liao ZC, Maestas R, Kirven LE, Eacker AM, Morales LS. Racial/ethnic disparities in clinical grading in medical school. Teach Learn Med. 2019;31(5):487–96. https://doi.org/10.1080/10401334.2019.1597724. Epub 2019 Apr 29. PMID: 31032666

Chapter 36
Maintenance of Certification (MOC), Continuing Medical Education (CME), and Conference Participation

Saifuddin T. Mama

After residency, the singular goal is passing the written and oral boards. In order to practice and obtain hospital privileges, you have to be board certified. The completion of the written and oral boards allows you to apply to become a fellow of the American College of Obstetricians and Gynecologists.

Initially after residency it will be easy to be distracted from accomplishing the goal of becoming board certified, whether it is due to being in fellowship training or starting your initial first attending job with all the attendant responsibilities.

Ideally, you should focus on completing both the written and oral boards as soon as feasible. This process has strict yearly deadlines for application so be aware of those in your planning.

Once you are boarded, to maintain the status of remaining board certified, you must participate in maintenance of certification (MOC). This is a requirement to remain board certified. It is in your employer's and your interest to remain board certified, so usually there is time allocated in the year to attend conferences and a stipend to pay for this as well as MOC and CME activities.

Concomitant with MOC is continuing medical education (CME). The goal of this process is providing a pathway for continuing to learn and to improve daily practice following initial certification.

For *maintenance of certification*, here is a link to the American Board of OBGYN (ABOG) portal.

ABOG—Physician Portal

Under my Media in the ABOG Portal are three tutorials with video links:

New ABOG Portal Tutorial: Diplomate Dashboard.
New ABOG Portal Tutorial: Lifelong Learning and Self-Assessment (Articles).

S. T. Mama (✉)
Division of Urogynecology, Department of Obstetrics and Gynecology, Cooper Medical School of Rowan University and Cooper University Health Care, Camden, NJ, USA

A. Malik et al. (eds.), *An Obstetrician/Gynecologist's Path*,
https://doi.org/10.1007/978-3-031-87098-9_36

New ABOG Portal Tutorial: Practice Improvement.

These tutorials provide supplemental information and clarification regarding the MOC process.

Steps required for MOC are as follows:

1. MOC Applications are available at the beginning of the year in January.
   This involves signing terms of agreement, including the following:
   - Details on clinical activity.
   - Specialty or subspecialty.
   - Percentage clinical effort.
   - Practice area of interest.
   - Options for applying for focused practice designation in either pediatric and adolescent gynecology (PAG) or minimally invasive gynecologic surgery (MIGS).
   - Active state medical license.
   - Active hospital privileges.
   - Board affiliations.
   - Attestation of professional standing, which includes details on the following:
     - Disciplinary action.
     - Misdemeanor or felonies.
     - Limitations, restrictions, suspension, revocation, resignation, investigation regarding privileges.
     - Conditions that impair judgment or conditions that adversely affect ability to practice medicine.
     - Required monitoring program mandated by licensing board.
     - Proctoring program mandated by hospital.
     - CME options.
     - Extra CME options.
2. Submission of self-nomination form/cover letter.
3. Submission of curriculum vitae.
4. Payment of administrative fee.
5. Completion of articles by Nov 15th of cycle year, with maintenance of score above 86% to stay on the performance pathway. Performance pathway allows the diplomat to maintain yearly certification without having to take a recertification exam.
6. Completion of practice improvement activities, one activity from available options below.
   - Modules—assessment, identification, and implementation of improvements in clinical practice, categories are MIGS, PAG, Urogynecology, Complex Family Planning, Gynecologic Oncology, Gynecology, Health Equity and Patient Safety, Maternal Fetal Medicine, Obstetrics, Office Practice, and Reproductive Endocrinology and Infertility.

An example of an activity within a category in Urogynecology—conservative management of pelvic organ prolapse, reading a short summary, then reviewing 10 patient charts in your practice.

- Quality improvement modules (40) or simulation modules (20).
- Posters, presentations, and publications focused on Quality Improvement (QI):
  - For posters and presentations, provide meeting program, date presented within MOC year, listed as author, clinical QI and not research, copy of poster with specific aim of Qi project, process for improvement, progress towards aim, discussion if aim achieved, related to diplomats practice content area.
  - For publication, publish in a peer-reviewed journal, adhere to SQUIRE guidelines, publish in the current MOC cycle, copy of publication, name of journal.
- Reciprocity—credit already received by another ABMS member board.
- Portfolio program—apply to sponsor QI or simulation study diplomate is leading.

At yearly completion of MOC, CME credits are automatically given.

Regardless of your position, whether in private practice or in an academic setting, there are minimum requirements yearly for CME. It is important to document Category 1 CME credits early. CME can take many forms. For any of these, you must check that there are Category 1 CME credits attached:

1. Completing MOC—this is focused on lifelong learning and practice improvement after obtaining board certification.
2. Signing up for additional articles to read and answer when completing MOC for extra CME credit.
3. Attending grand rounds.
4. Attending morbidity and mortality conference.
5. Attending conferences.
6. Attending hospital-based workshop/meeting/conferences.
7. Attending industry base workshop/meeting/conferences.

The institution you're at may keep electronic records for grand rounds and other educational activities providing category 1 CME credits; otherwise, you have to keep track and record your hours. In the same manner that you keep your curriculum vitae updated, make it a habit monthly to update your category 1 CME credits. For conference activity, keep in mind that credits are only applied after you have filled out the evaluations. It is best to complete these as soon as the conference is over or after each day at the conference. It is a good habit to print out the certificates as soon as they are completed and keep a folder for the year.

Conferences serve many purposes: selecting conferences is based on your goals.

1. Validation of knowledge and practice within your field.
2. Exposure to new knowledge in your field or other related fields.

3. Exposure to new procedures.
4. Exposure to new technology.
5. Opportunity to meet established experts in the field.
6. Opportunity to become involved at the regional and national level. Many areas for service exist, such as volunteering for a committee in your area of interest; serving on the scientific committee or abstract committee in preparation for annual conferences; and serving as a liaison to other organizations or representing the needs of the society at the local, state, and national levels in order to effect change.
7. Opportunity for colleagues you know to introduce you to their network of colleagues.
8. Opportunity to meet colleagues with similar academic interests to initiate joint multicenter research projects.
9. Joint publications with other colleagues.
10. Presenting at regional, national, or international conferences, either poster, oral, workshops, or symposiums as part of your academic duties and to be able to connect with colleagues working on similar academic pursuits.

As a new graduate, first pick conferences based on your academic interests and what you find compelling. Equally important is to choose conferences and preconference workshops based on an awareness of gaps in your knowledge. While you're doing this, make a serious effort to meet attendees with similar interests. Attend morning or lunchtime roundtables, which present a more intimate setting to get to know other attendees. Do not be afraid to go up to known experts in the field, especially with questions and cases you don't know the answer to. After scientific sessions, feel free to go up to speakers with questions. Most speakers at all levels are very willing to converse with you. Attend all receptions for new attendees as these are designed to help you feel comfortable and feel part of the conference. As you continue to network and attend conferences within the realm of your special interests, you will get to know many more people outside your institution. As early as possible, look for opportunities to present research, case studies, or protocols at conferences—this will help you attract like-minded people and continue to build your professional network.

After the initial phase of establishing your practice and board certification, you will continue to learn and grow. Use required MOC, CME, and conferences to your advantage, and you will quickly find an ever-expanding knowledge base and network of colleagues.

Chapter 37
Board Exams

Lori Adriance

You've completed four years of medical school, four years of residency training, passed three board exams, taken multiple in-service exams, and are finally graduating as an obstetrician gynecologist. But wait, you're still not done! Board certification is the final step in this journey. For obstetrics and gynecology, board certification is a two-step process including the qualifying exam followed by the certifying exam, or more commonly referred to as the written and oral exams, respectively.

As of 2020, graduates also need to pass a Surgical Skills Program to be eligible for American Board of Obstetrics and Gynecology (ABOG) certification. As of this writing, this means you must achieve either Essentials in Minimally Invasive Gynecologic Surgery (EMIGS) or Fundamentals of Laparoscopic Surgery (FLS) certification to be eligible to move forward as an Active Candidate for Ob/Gyn certification.

The qualifying exam is offered annually as the first of two exams required for board certification in obstetrics and gynecology. The exam traditionally takes place in July after graduation and must be taken in person at a Pearson VUE Testing Center. It is scheduled to last 3 hours and 45 minutes and will assess your knowledge in obstetrics and gynecology, as well as the subspecialties of maternal fetal medicine, urogynecology, gynecologic oncology, and reproductive endocrinology. The exam consists of 230 single-best answer, multiple-choice questions. The results of the qualifying exam will be reported online to each candidate on or before the last Friday in October.

Once you have passed the qualifying exam, you are now eligible to take the certifying exam, which tends to be the more intimidating of the two. The certifying exam takes place in person, at ABOG headquarters in Dallas, Texas. It consists of

L. Adriance (✉)
Department of Obstetrics and Gynecology, Cooper Medical School of Rowan University and Cooper University Health Care, Camden, NJ, USA

A. Malik et al. (eds.), *An Obstetrician/Gynecologist's Path*,
https://doi.org/10.1007/978-3-031-87098-9_37

three parts: obstetrics, gynecology, and office practice. Each part lasts 1 hour each, with 30 minutes dedicated to structured cases and 30 minutes dedicated to your case list. There are two examiners per candidate in each section.

Per ABOG, case lists must include all patients primarily cared for by the candidate where the candidate holds privileges between July 1st and June 30th of the same academic year. The lists must include a minimum of 20 obstetrical and 20 gynecological admissions, but all patients must be listed. This includes all patients admitted as well as all short-stay and outpatient surgical patients, even if not officially admitted to a hospital. The case list must demonstrate sufficient number, breadth, and depth of clinical experience. If a candidate does not have a minimum of 20 cases for obstetrics or gynecology, a candidate may use an 18-month case list and/or an appropriate number of cases from fellowship or senior residency case logs. However, candidates may not use senior resident or prior fellowship cases to meet minimum numbers for both the obstetrics and gynecology case lists. The office practice case list is strictly limited to 40 patients with conditions that fit into the listed office practice categories available on the ABOG website. Candidates may not reuse any case or case list from a previous examination. The list(s) of obstetrics and gynecology patients from each hospital and surgical center must be verified on the Case List Affidavit form. The records librarian or similar hospital official must complete the Case List Affidavit Form attesting that all hospitalized or surgical center patients primarily cared for by the candidate are listed for the period indicated. The list of patients provided by the candidate is subject to independent verification and audit by an agent or employee of ABOG.

Of note, a candidate must achieve board certification within eight years of completing residency. If more than eight years have elapsed since the completion of residency training, a candidate is no longer eligible to apply for either the qualifying or certifying exams until they have completed a minimum of 6 months of supervised practice at a hospital affiliated with an ACGME-accredited training program. Years spent in ACGME-accredited fellowship or a secondary residency do not count towards the eight-year limit.

While all of this sounds, and frankly is, quite daunting, it is all about preparation. The goal of board certification is to verify you are a competent and safe obstetrician and gynecologist. Half of the certifying exam is your own case list, which means you control half of the exam (to a certain extent). This means you want to make sure your list is accurate, aesthetically pleasing (meaning easy to read for the examiners), and contains just the right amount of detail to help you remember the patient without giving too much away. Your case list is not the time for the zebras. It does not need to be "interesting," just complete. Have your case list reviewed, whether it be mentors from your residency program, your current job, or a professional company. Once it is submitted, you cannot change it! After submitting, it is important to know your case list well, as half of the exam will come straight from what you provided.

Just like any other board exam, it is, of course, important to study and know the medical information. However, this is not the place for the latest and greatest trials. This will not impress the examiners. Stick to ACOG practice bulletins and committee opinions, foundational textbooks, and the landmark trials. Unfortunately, many great physicians who have failed their oral boards have not done so due to lack of knowledge, but rather inability to articulate their knowledge to the examiners in a high-stress situation. I recall being "voluntold" to participate in a mock oral exam at a preparation course. In front of hundreds of my colleagues, I could not recall the ingredients in the birth control pill I prescribe regularly. The panic and embarrassment set in, and my mind went blank. After what felt like hours of torture, I was finally dismissed back to my seat. Of course, as soon as I returned to my chair, I recalled all of the answers. Do not let this happen on exam day. You need to practice. I highly recommend exam courses, webinars, and mock orals. Practice verbally articulating your answers and thought process. The more you practice answering out loud, the more likely this will feel like second nature on exam day. Also know that the examiners will push you with their questioning to the point that you do not know. That's ok. Don't make it up. Admit you would need to look it up. Give the safe answer. Remember, the examiners want to verify that you are a competent and safe obstetrician and gynecologist. You are. You just need to show them.

Chapter 38
Medical Economics

Joseph Maccarone

The Maze of Medical Economics

Congratulations! You are beginning your journey as an Ob/Gyn attending, be it as part of a health system or as a private practitioner. You went into medicine wanting to help all individuals who walked through your door, regardless of the monetary incentives at the end of the day. Nevertheless, though we attempt to avoid the topic, there is no denying the financial implications of the delivery of care.

According to CMS data from 2022, the national healthcare expenditure in the United States amounted to $4.5 trillion, or $13,493 per person, up 4.1% from the previous year. This represented 17.3% of the GDP. By 2031, healthcare spending is predicted to outpace average GDP growth, resulting in its share of the GDP increasing to 19.6% [8]. At the same time, healthcare outcomes are not reflected in this increased spending. The maternal mortality rate was the highest among similar countries at 23.8 deaths per 100,000 live births in 2020, compared to the average of 3.6 deaths per 100,000 live births. Moreover, the US also possessed the highest infant mortality rate (5.4 deaths per 1000 live births), the second highest rate of obstetric trauma during vaginal delivery (11.7 per 100 births), and consistently higher cesarean sections (317.9 per 1000 live births vs. an average of 264.3 per 1000 live births in comparable countries) [5].

From these statistics, it is impossible to ignore the economic impact of healthcare. Medicine is, for better or worse, a business whose viability is paramount to be able to care for all populations. When institutions are no longer able to maintain

J. Maccarone (✉)
Georgetown University, Washington, DC, USA

Cooper Medical School of Rowan University, Camden, NJ, USA

A. Malik et al. (eds.), *An Obstetrician/Gynecologist's Path*,
https://doi.org/10.1007/978-3-031-87098-9_38

profitability, care delivery is compromised, staff lose their jobs, and providers shut their doors.

Simply put, patients suffer.

So how do we decipher the complex labyrinth of medical economics to ensure not only our financial viability and continuous improvement but also serve as advocates for our patients as they too navigate the system? How can we improve the delivery of quality, affordable healthcare and bolster outcomes while simultaneously cutting costs?

Let's strap in, and, fair warning, this is going to get bumpy.

Medical Economics: Where to Begin?

Picture this: you are 17 again, a newly printed license with the ink barely dry, and a set of keys to the rusty Toyota Camry that has been passed down from sibling to sibling. Sliding behind the wheel, you are excited to turn that key and gain your freedom as you hit the open road.

But wait! You realize in dismay that you have not signed up for car insurance. So, you go online, pull up a quote, and proceed to fall out of your chair at the multitude of zeros emanating from the screen. With a sigh of dismay, you sign up, print out your insurance card, and away you go.

For those of us who have had the fortune (and at times misfortune) of owning a car, we know one of the requirements that can come in the form of insurance fees, designed to protect not only us but other individuals in the case of an accident. It is a requirement to own a car and often a barrier for countless individuals. As a result, some may try to risk it: driving uninsured and hoping they don't get pulled over, or worse, be the victim of a costly and life-altering accident.

Yet, while we set requirements on insurance for automobiles to safeguard against the unforeseeable, the same does not apply to health insurance. The Individual Mandate, a component of the Affordable Care Act (ACA), attempted to correct this but was ultimately repealed in 2019 by the Supreme Court. The result is that every one of us is granted the autonomy, for better or for worse, to determine what level of health coverage we will choose each year.

This brings us to the core of this chapter: what motivates some individuals to gain comprehensive health insurance, high-deductible health plans, or choose to live without it entirely? What fuels the exponential rise in healthcare costs, and how do supply and demand factor in? And how can we as providers work to curb healthcare spending through rational clinical decision-making? Let's dive in.

The History of Health Insurance

In the early days of medicine, physicians made house calls and accepted goods and services from those they cared for as payment. Over time, the culture of bartering became monetary payments, with individuals paying out of pocket for every aspect of care they received. As you can imagine, this meant that healthcare had become more and more cost-prohibitive for the masses. It was not until 1929, at the dawn of the Great Depression, that the insurance we know today was conceived at Baylor University Hospital. Referred to as the "Baylor Plan," this plan guaranteed Dallas teachers 21 days in the hospital annually for the low cost of 50 cents per month (equivalent to approximately 7 dollars today) [3]. Just like that, the first employer-sponsored health plan was born and would go on to become Blue Cross today. Today, employer-sponsored health insurance remains the most common subtype, covering 54.5% of those insured in the United States or approximately 180 million individuals [4].

The Basics of Health Insurance: A Crash Course in Costs

To talk about health insurance requires defining basic terms, such as premium, deductible, and co-pay. A "premium" is the monthly fee paid to the insurance company, which varies based on age, ZIP code, competition between insurance agencies, smoking status, and the type of plan. The "deductible," on the other hand, can be seen as the threshold of out-of-pocket costs that must be reached before insurance kicks in and pays the rest. For those with "high-deductible health plans," or HDHP, individuals have a lower premium with the condition that they are responsible for a higher percentage of their medical expenditures in the case of an emergency. In these cases, individuals are encouraged to store money in a Health Savings Account (HSA), which is a tax-advantaged account designed to pay for medical expenditures not covered by insurance. Finally, we have "co-pays," the specified dollar amount you pay when receiving a specific type of service. These vary by setting of care: for example, a primary care visit may cost $15, while an ER visit may cost as much as $200 due to the level of care received in this setting.

While I could spend 20 pages talking about the many nuances of insurance, you're now equipped with the rudimentary concepts to get you through the next question: what does it have to do with medical economics?

Risk and Risk Aversion

Doubt is not a pleasant condition, but certainty is absurd—Voltaire [2].

Risk is present in every aspect of our lives: applying to our dream medical school or residency programs, asking a crush on a date, or investing in a new business pursuit. In all of these cases, we are trading our time, ability, and/or monetary resources against the risk of failure. Some risks are more unconscious, woven into the fabric of our day-to-day existence. For example, we may choose to ride our bike to work without thinking of the inherent risk of being in an accident. We (begrudgingly) forego sleep or healthy food choices at times on call to care for patients or study for an exam, knowing it may catch up to us later.

But how do we determine what risk is acceptable, and what is beyond what we are comfortable with?

This brings us to the concept of risk aversion: the tendency to pick a situation that is highly predictable but with a lower payoff as opposed to a highly unpredictable one with a potentially higher payoff. Risk aversion is present not only in economics (do you choose to put your money in a bank or stocks), but also in everyday life. If you are willing to ride your bike to work, then what about a motorcycle? Most doctors would reflect on the amount of motorcycle-involved MVAs they've seen in the trauma bay and opt for a safer form of transportation. Nevertheless, millions of Americans ride motorcycles every day (some of whom are your very colleagues and the author of this chapter).

The same principles apply to healthcare and insurance. We often think of it through a cost-benefit analysis (CBA). Does the potential cost of riding a motorcycle (maintenance, insurance, and the risk of bodily injury and/or death) outweigh the benefit (the thrill of the open road, stress management, "coolness" factor)? Does the cost of health insurance (usually monetary) outweigh the benefit (minimal out-of-pocket costs for office visits, prescriptions, and/or medical emergencies requiring hospitalization)?

Those who are younger and healthier are typically more risk "tolerant" and willing to forego the costly, comprehensive health insurance plans in favor of high-deductible health plans, which place responsibility on the individual to save in a health savings account (HSA), or no coverage at all. On the other end of the spectrum, a middle-aged man with several chronic medical conditions will prefer a comprehensive plan with little out-of-pocket costs.

While this seems simple enough, healthcare does not occur in a vacuum. Next, we will explore some of the problems associated with insurance coverage, as well as the utilization of healthcare resources.

Adverse Selection: Fostering an Unsustainable Insurance Marketplace

Insurance companies, like any business venture, are concerned with being profitable. How do they do this in the realm of healthcare? While they employ complex algorithms to determine premiums based on the consumer, one simple aspect is the employment of "risk pools." The assumption is that a relatively large portion of insurance holders will be in "good" health, thereby resulting in low utilization of healthcare resources in a given year. In contrast, a small percentage of insured individuals will fall into the "high utilizer" category, accounting for the majority of healthcare spending. By pooling large numbers of healthy individuals with these high utilizers, insurance companies can minimize the cost impact of these individuals. However, while this occurs in all industries, there are several problems associated with risk pooling in health insurance.

The individual mandate, by compelling all individuals to be covered or face penalties, was one attempt to curb the principle of adverse selection: when either buyers or sellers have information that the other party does not. In healthcare, this is usually the individual seeking insurance, who has information regarding their health that insurance companies do not possess. Likewise, with the stipulation in the ACA that insurance companies cannot deny coverage based on preexisting conditions, we see a large number of high-utilizers entering the marketplace. In contrast, healthy individuals may choose HDHPs or no insurance at all. This relates to the cost-benefit analysis (CBA) we all undergo in every aspect of our lives: we will only seek insurance when the benefit of coverage outweighs the (financial) cost.

Consequently, adverse selection results in risk pools composed of a significant percentage of high-utilizers and insufficient healthy, low-utilizers. Such a pool would be unprofitable for insurers, forcing them to raise premiums to ensure their bottom line is intact. Yet, in doing so, more individuals will reevaluate their CBAs, resulting in a fraction exiting the market as they deem insurance to be too costly. In response, insurance companies raise their premiums, more insured individuals leave the market, insurers raise their premiums…

Do you see where I am going with this?

As businesses will only remain if they deem the market a "profitable" entity, this questions the future sustainability of privatized systems amidst rising costs and offers one benefit of a socialized system with universal coverage seen in other nations.

Moral Hazard and Consumer-Driven Health Care: Don't Be Afraid to Take Risks! It's Covered…

Moral hazard is another principle that works hand in hand with adverse selection and is thought to increase healthcare utilization. It refers to the concept that, by bearing a smaller out-of-pocket stake in their medical costs, individuals are likely to consume more care and demand more costly care, fail to engage in preventive behavior or engage in unhealthy and/or risky behaviors, and lack the incentive to search for and demand lower healthcare costs. One method to curb overutilization is through gatekeepers, such as PCPs, who require prior authorization for specialty visits. Co-payments and deductibles are also employed as financial deterrents, compelling individuals to use resources appropriately.

In reality, the concept of moral hazard has been met with mixed results and is often an overutilized justification for increasing healthcare costs. By its logic, socialized systems should reveal extreme overutilization of resources without financial disincentives. Yet, health expenditures per person in the US were double that spent in comparable countries ($12,555 vs $6651) [9].

This has prompted the push toward "Consumer-Driven Health Care" to empower individuals to take control of their health decisions and spending. Through the use of high-deductible health plans and health savings accounts, individuals are incentivized to engage in preventive care and healthy behaviors that limit the high costs of secondary and tertiary care structures while being acutely aware of healthcare costs and spending. Still, this concept is riddled with problems innate to healthcare as a "commodity" and transforms a systemic problem into an individual burden.

Achieving Equitable, Adequate Coverage

According to KFF data from 2022, 25.6 million Americans remain uninsured, the majority of whom are adults, in low-income families, and people of color [7]. These individuals represent the longstanding rift between qualifying for federally sponsored health care (Medicaid, especially in states that have opted against Medicaid expansion) and being able to afford a plan on the healthcare marketplace with their limited resources. In a nutshell: too poor to afford to purchase care, but too "rich" to qualify for federally sponsored care. These statistics do not begin to include the millions of undocumented noncitizens living in the United States who would likewise benefit from insurance coverage but are consistently barred from taking part in federal programs.

However, in our fight to close the deep-rooted insurance chasm, we forget about an issue that is not as "flashy": the millions who are not uninsured but rather *underinsured*. Remember those HDHPs mentioned in this chapter? Regrettably, they are a big perpetrator of this reality. Faced with prohibitive out-of-pocket costs and a lack of sufficient savings, individuals and families may forgo needed prescriptions to manage their chronic conditions. As a result, there is an overutilization of costly, tertiary care structures. This shows the nature of a "reactive" system of medicine, instead of one that could proactively curb costs through widespread, equitable, and accessible coverage.

FFS vs. VBC

To understand healthcare reimbursements as a provider, it is important to have a rudimentary understanding of the history of payment models and their role, for better or worse, in healthcare decision-making.

Historically, healthcare operated under a Fee-For-Service (FFS) model, which reimbursed providers for each service they delivered, regardless of outcome. This incentivized providers to provide more and more complex services, driving up quantity with little emphasis on the actual quality of care. As you can imagine, this reimbursement method was not always met with the best intentions. Hospital stays for routine procedures were excessive, as providers were able to bill for each day they retained the patient. Uncomplicated vaginal births, while averaging 24–48 hour hospital stays today, could be as long as 4 days or more [1]. Likewise, there was no incentive towards preventive care, but rather secondary and tertiary care structures with higher billables.

Faced with gross overutilization of resources, the national health expenditure soared to incredible heights, placing pressure on a faltering system to devise new payment methods to curb inflation. This led to the introduction of Value-based Care (VBC) models, aimed at curbing utilization, increasing efficiency and quality of care, and improving health outcomes. Instead of being paid per procedure, institutions are provided bundled payments. Therefore, for each episode of care, they are paid a fixed, single payment regardless of the services delivered. For the first time, providers now have a level of shared financial risk with insurers: to be profitable, they must work to curb costs below set reimbursements and achieve quality and performance metrics. This incentivizes efficiency and quality of care by emphasizing cost-effective preventive care to avoid chronic illness and reliance on costly secondary and tertiary care structures, limit unnecessary tests, and curb length-of-stay in hospitalizations. At the same time, by linking reimbursements to process, quality, and efficiency measures, institutions are financially incentivized towards continuous quality improvement and employment of "best practice" approaches to care.

While this is a promising direction for healthcare reimbursement, barriers to adoption, such as added responsibility on providers, allow FFS to continue as a predominant payment model for provider services.

Supply and Demand of Healthcare

Turning back to the story at the beginning of the chapter: you are 17 again, now with insurance, and have finally been able to drive that rusty Toyota to school each day. Several months go by without a hitch, and though you can barely scrape enough together for gas money and insurance payments, life is finally looking up. One hot summer day, you are sitting in traffic when smoke begins emanating from the engine compartment. 3 hours and a mechanic visit later, you are staring at a $500 bill for a new radiator. How are you ever going to afford it? With a look of resignation, you opt to return to biking for the foreseeable future until you finally save up enough to repair the car.

Our bodies are much like the cars on the road every single day: forced to start and stop, regulate a thousand different parameters to maintain optimal temperature and functioning capacity, and prone to malfunction at a moment's notice. When things go wrong, we find ourselves in the primary care office, or worse, in the ED.

However, this is where the comparison ends.

What we often don't realize is that health is a "commodity," just as much as the cars we drive, the houses we live in, the food we eat, and any other items we may purchase. However, when it comes to healthcare, the economic principles of supply and demand differ significantly from other goods and services.

First, let's define supply and demand:

Supply refers to the availability of healthcare resources, either within a specific market or health system. This can include facilities (such as hospitals, outpatient offices, and labs), medical equipment, pharmaceuticals, staff (physicians, nurses, techs), and other resources paramount to the delivery of services.

Demand, on the other hand, is the desire and/or willingness of individuals to seek care depending on the price of doing so (ultimately their ability to pay for it given certain income restraints). Economics assumes that consumers will purchase goods that maximize their "utility" (satisfaction or benefit derived from consuming a good or service) [6].

Now, let's unpack how they differ in medical economics:

Unlike most goods, healthcare is a "derived demand," meaning it does not directly affect utility. (Instead, the demand for care is brought about by the demand for good health: we seek care to maintain our health or improve it when we are sick. An easy example of this is seen in smartphones. Demand for smartphones may be driven by various factors such as consumer preferences, increased communication, and new features. At the same time, these devices cannot be made without lithium-ion batteries. In this scenario, the demand for lithium-ion batteries serves as the "derived demand." Just as the increase in demand for lithium-ion batteries is indirectly driven by the demand for smartphones, so is the demand for healthcare resources indirectly driven by the demand for good health.

Moreover, healthcare supply and demand are considered inelastic. This means that, regardless of changes to the quantity or price of services, it will have minimal impact on the supply or demand of healthcare services, respectively.

On the supply side, healthcare rarely possesses the scalable infrastructure to increase supply quickly enough to meet increasing demand. This revolves around limited existing infrastructure, time constraints, and an increasing shortage of healthcare professionals, among other factors. A recent example is the COVID-19 pandemic, where demand rose at an exponential rate while supply struggled to increase at a proportional rate (such as in facility space, personnel, and PPE).

On the demand side, when consumers seek medical care, it is not always at their discretion. When our car breaks down, we have the luxury of obtaining quotes from various mechanics to find the highest quality at the lowest price. In contrast, when a medical emergency occurs, all opportunities to "shop around" are instantly thrown out the window in favor of the nearest facility equipped to handle our specific condition. Indeed, we are consistently faced with limited alternatives in healthcare, regardless of the costs, from the insulin-dependent diabetic to the expectant mother requiring an unplanned c-section. The "life-saving" nature of care often leads to an increased tolerance of wait times (such as waiting for multiple hours in the ED or months for an appointment) and the short/long-term costs of care, regardless of how debilitating they may be. Just as health outcomes are known to vastly change between zip codes, so can demand and utilization in response to factors such as population demographics, the prevalence of health conditions, income and socioeconomic status, insurance coverage, accessibility, cultural and social factors, and health education, among others.

An Unwelcome Surprise: The Reality of Healthcare Billing

Complicated enough? Sadly, there is one more complexity to discuss in medical economics: a lack of price transparency that prohibits patients, providers, and payers alike from curtailing rising costs. If you have ever received a medical bill, you can recall the anxiety-provoking complexity of each line item spelled out, from the facility fees, providers' fees, equipment, and medications, to the insurance negotiations and reimbursement rate. What remains is a final number obscured in a plethora of billing codes and financial negotiations between health systems and insurance companies.

For those who have ever looked closely at these itemized lists, they contain truly staggering examples of inflated costs, such as 60 dollars for an ibuprofen or a simple bandage (which can be procured at a drug store in a large quantity for only a few bucks). But who pays for the $60 ibuprofen on the bill? The patient? The insurance provider? The hospital?

The true answer will surprise you: no one.

No one? Yes, you heard that right: the price shown on the bill is part of a larger bargaining game between healthcare systems and insurance companies over their rates of reimbursement. Depending on the insurance type, healthcare systems may only be reimbursed a fraction of the actual costs outlined in the bill. For example, Medicaid and Medicare may reimburse hospitals approximately 20–25 and 80–85 cents, respectively, for every dollar spent on a patient's care. Unfortunately, hospitals have to remain profitable and often deal with this underpayment through their negotiations with private insurance companies. This depends heavily on the bargaining power of hospitals, aka their leverage to negotiate higher reimbursement rates for items such as ibuprofen or a bandage. Hospitals that serve as the primary or lone provider for a geographic area, offer high-quality and cutting-edge services, and have a high patient volume will have the largest bargaining power. Likewise, the amount of insurance providers in the region plays a role, as increased competition can promote more favorable rates as insurance providers seek to expand their provider networks against rival companies.

In the end, this is one of the predominant reasons for the discrepancies in cost for identical procedures between hospitals. A hospital with low bargaining power and a subsequently low reimbursement rate may set higher costs for ibuprofen to offset their costs. As a result, the price is reduced to a markedly less shocking amount by the end of insurance adjustments.

This brings us to one of our last topics: surprise billing and balance billing. Surprise billing, or surprise out-of-network billing, occurs when care is delivered by a provider outside of the patient's insurance network, typically without their consent or knowledge. Patients are only aware of the occurrence when they receive a substantial bill that insurance refuses to cover. Balanced billing is a similar occurrence, in that providers bill patients for the difference that remains following insurance reimbursement and what the provider charges, instead of accepting the insurance reimbursement as payment in full. Today, state and federal legislation, such as the "No Surprises Act," is rapidly curbing these billing practices and hopefully lessening the financial strain on vulnerable populations.

Conclusion: A System Doomed to Fail?

In conclusion, the field of medical economics plays a crucial role in understanding some of the many factors that influence the day-to-day operations and viability of the healthcare industry. Throughout this chapter, we have outlined key aspects of medical economics, including what draws individuals to purchase insurance and seek care, the changing landscape of healthcare reimbursements, the problems with traditional supply and demand principles in healthcare, and finally the tumultuous reality of healthcare billing.

So, what does this mean for you as providers?

While this chapter may have painted a bleak landscape of escalating costs and an unsustainable system, there is a glimmer of hope for the future. As key stakeholders in the medical system, it will be up to you as Ob/Gyn providers to effectively and efficiently manage healthcare delivery, promote patient education, engage in advocacy efforts, navigate the complexities of billing and reimbursement, and focus on continuous quality improvement efforts. It is in this way that providers can serve as crucial leaders at the forefront of medical economics, to help shape a sustainable, high-quality healthcare system that delivers equitable care for generations to come.

Works Cited

1. Backes EP, Scrimshaw SC, editors. Birth settings in America: outcomes, quality, access, and choice. Washington, DC: National Academies Press; 2020.
2. Encyclopædia Britannica, Inc. Voltaire: Quotes. Encyclopædia Britannica. 2024. https://www.britannica.com/quotes/Voltaire
3. Gorman L. The history of health care costs and health insurance. Wisconsin Policy Research Institute Rep. 2006;19(10):1–31.

4. Keisler-Starkey K, Bunch L, Lindstrom R., Health Insurance Coverage in the United States: 2022. United States Census Bureau. 2023. Retrieved April 2024, from https://www.census.gov/content/dam/Census/library/publications/2023/demo/p60-281.pdf
5. OECD. Health status (Edition 2020). OECD Health Statistics (database). 2021. https://doi.org/10.1787/321b42dd-en. Accessed on 06 May 2024.
6. Rodriguez Santana I, Mason A, Gutacker N, Kasteridis P, Santos R, Rice N. Need, demand, supply in health care: working definitions, and their implications for defining access. Health Econ Policy Law. 2023;18(1):1–13. https://doi.org/10.1017/S1744133121000293.
7. Tolbert J, Drake P, Damico A. Key Facts about the Uninsured Population. KFF. 2023, December 18. https://www.kff.org/uninsured/issue-brief/key-facts-about-the-uninsured-population/
8. U.S. Centers for Medicare & Medicaid Services. NHE Fact Sheet. 2023, December 13. CMS.gov. https://www.cms.gov/data-research/statistics-trends-and-reports/national-health-expenditure-data/nhe-fact-sheet
9. Wager E, McGough M, Rakshit S, Amin K, Cox C. How does health spending in the U.S. compare to other countries?. Peterson-KFF Health System Tracker. 2024, January 23. https://www.healthsystemtracker.org/chart-collection/health-spending-u-s-compare-countries/#GDP%20per%20capita%20and%20health%20consumption%20spending%20per%20capita,%202022%20(U.S.%20dollars,%20PPP%20adjusted

Chapter 39
Medical Ethics

Joseph Maccarone

Every provider remembers a pivotal moment in their medical education: their white coat ceremony, where they donned their first short coats and recited the Hippocratic Oath in front of loved ones. This longstanding oath, which has grown and changed since its inception, is not merely a symbolic ritual but rather a moral compass to uphold the highest ethical standards in healthcare practice. It marks the first time you pledged to serve patients with integrity and compassion, promoting their well-being throughout the continuum of care.

As Ob/Gyn providers, you are entrusted with a special responsibility not seen in other medical disciplines, encompassing a wide spectrum of well-being and reproductive health. From routine exams to cancer screenings, prenatal care, family planning and contraception, reproductive health education, and gynecologic surgery, there are countless roles you will serve in guiding the populations within your care through critical life milestones that will shape their very identities.

What you may come to realize, however, is that the reality of clinical medicine rarely parallels the succinct, black-and-white answers seen in any textbook or board exam. In fact, medicine often forces us as providers to defy our nature of seeking comfort in certainty, the black and white, and allow ourselves instead to be uncomfortable living within the large swaths of uncertainty, the "gray," that permeate our very existence. An important aspect of care in this realm is the ethical decisions that are interwoven within clinical decision-making, which require empathetic listening, thoughtful reflection, and a basic understanding of the principles of medical ethics.

In our modern world, this responsibility has only grown in importance, as we witness a nation divided over reproductive rights.

J. Maccarone (✉)
Georgetown University, Washington, DC, USA

Cooper Medical School of Rowan University, Camden, NJ, USA

A. Malik et al. (eds.), *An Obstetrician/Gynecologist's Path*,
https://doi.org/10.1007/978-3-031-87098-9_39

Across this chapter, we will delve into the principles of autonomy, beneficence, nonmaleficence, and justice and explore how they fit into the realm of Ob/Gyn care. We will also illuminate many of the complexities within decision-making and how providers can approach novel ethical dilemmas head-on as they arise.

History of Medical Ethics: Lost Trust in the Medical Field

The history of medicine, contrary to the pure, pristine image of the white coat we wear, is sullied by the ethical transgressions committed under the guise of "progress" or "medical innovation". Medical experiments were routinely conducted on vulnerable populations without adequate protection or informed consent, such as prisoners, minorities, people with disabilities, women, children, and displaced populations. Indeed, some of the most celebrated discoveries and physicians in history were made in this way. For example, Walter Reed, a U.S. Army physician whose name has adorned "Walter Reed National Military Medical Center" since its inception, established the transmission of yellow fever by the Aedes aegypti mosquito during the Spanish-American War. This medical breakthrough came at the expense of countless ethical violations, including a lack of informed consent, coercion of soldiers and locals, and an extreme risk of harm to the participants. Though time went on, the transgressions continued: Nazi medical experiments in World War II, the Tuskegee Syphilis Study from 1932 to 1972, Henrietta Lacks in 1951, and the case of Baby Doe in 1982 [6].

While these are not all-encompassing, each transgression further sowed the deep-seated mistrust and skepticism towards medicine that persists to this day. It is through employing the ethical principles discussed in this chapter that we can work towards rebuilding this trust in this generation.

Roe v. Wade: A Shot Heard Round the World for Reproductive Rights

In order to talk about medical ethics, we first must delve into one of the most consequential pieces of legislation on healthcare today: *Roe v. Wade.*

Roe v. Wade, passed in 1973, legalized abortion nationwide and solidified reproductive rights as fundamental human rights. It reinforced the importance of safeguarding individual autonomy, the principle that a person has the right to make decisions about their own body, such as carrying or terminating a pregnancy. Furthermore, it marked an important step in reinforcing patient-centered care, as it affirmed healthcare decisions based on the needs and values of the patient above all other considerations.

However, this all came crashing down in 2022, when *Roe v. Wade* was overturned by the Supreme Court after nearly 50 years. The impact on the healthcare system was immediate: states began enforcing abortion bans and enacting legislation against both patients and providers who engaged in these services. These bans not only forced individuals to attempt and seek care out of state but also led to an increase in adverse outcomes due to their often political, and not medically based, origins. Providers feared providing emergency abortions even in cases of ectopic pregnancies, for fear of legal ramifications. While bans came to outline life-saving exceptions, the enduring nebulousness continues to create delays and reduce access to timely medical care. This may lead to current and future providers choosing to practice in states with less restrictive health policies. As a result, it calls into question not only the future of patient autonomy in reproductive health but also the availability of Ob/Gyn providers in states with strict abortion bans.

As we navigate the foundational principles of medical ethics in the next paragraphs, take the time to reflect on how they relate to cases such as *Roe v. Wade*.

Autonomy

Autonomy refers to an individual's right to make informed decisions regarding their healthcare, based on their specific needs, values, and goals. A key element of this is informed consent, where patients should be provided with all relevant information about their medical condition(s), treatment options, and the potential risks and benefits of these interventions. Yet, many of our patients do not have the medical backgrounds to make such decisions at face value. It is the role of medical providers to aid in this understanding by distilling the complexity of medical jargon into plain language and then checking understanding with methods such as the "teach-back," where a patient explains in their own words what they now know. This process must be unbiased and free from coercion, regardless of the outcome the patient may choose. While we tend to think of it in terms of informed consent, it also pertains to the realm of informed refusal, where a patient may knowingly refuse a potentially life-saving intervention. Even if we disagree with such choices, our job lies in helping patients understand potential consequences and upholding their right to refuse treatment. Today, healthcare has made great strides in upholding patients' wishes, such as through advanced directives and POLST (Physician Orders for Life-Sustaining Treatment) forms. A final aspect we will cover in autonomy lies in a patient's right to privacy and confidentiality of their health information and interactions. Through HIPAA (health insurance portability and accountability Act) privacy and security rulings, it is not only an ethical consideration but also a legal mandate to safeguard patient information and share it with only authorized individuals.

Beneficence

Beneficence relates to the obligation of healthcare providers to act in the best interests of their patients to promote their well-being. This goes beyond the principle of nonmaleficence, doing no harm, to actively helping others and maximizing the benefit to those within your care. As a provider, this will require you to engage in evidence-based medicine, utilizing your clinical expertise alongside current best-practice approaches to craft individualized treatment options for patients. This is seen in many aspects of Ob/Gyn care. Through comprehensive, proactive prenatal care, providers can promote the well-being of the pregnant individual and fetus while detecting complications early to minimize the risk of adverse outcomes. During labor and delivery, this involves monitoring labor, pain management, and rapid intervention to address complications such as fetal distress or maternal hemorrhage. In the realm of reproductive health, contraceptive counseling, and family planning can help empower individuals to make informed decisions, support reproductive autonomy, and reduce unintended pregnancies. In light of reproductive health issues, empathetic care and counseling can help address not only the physical but social and emotional health of the patient as well.

Nonmaleficence

Primum non nocere: First, do no harm [5].

In the realm of Ob/Gyn care, where you may be tasked with treating not only the individual but also an unborn child, nonmaleficence is of utmost importance. While beneficence calls on providers to act in ways to maximize benefit to the patient, nonmaleficence calls on us to minimize risk and harm to the best of our ability. An example within prenatal care is the utilization of screening/diagnostic tests. Invasive tests, such as amniocentesis or CVS, carry with them a small risk of complications and miscarriage in 1:200 cases [3]. Therefore, these tests are only considered when the potential benefit of the findings, such as the identification of a potentially lethal genetic condition, outweighs these risks. Even with the advent of noninvasive modalities, such as cfDNA screening, the process of testing still carries risks for increased stress and anxiety, as well as potential false positives [2]. In labor and delivery, the principle of nonmaleficence is seen in the medical indications for c-sections and the efforts to reduce unnecessary and elective procedures nationwide. Though they can be life-saving, c-sections have also been associated with increased maternal morbidity and mortality, increased recovery, postoperative complications, and an impact on future pregnancies. Providers must account for evidence-based practices, individual risk factors, and shared decision-making with the patient to promote positive outcomes for both the mother and child.

Justice

Justice pertains to the equitable, fair, and appropriate allocation of healthcare resources and the treatment of individuals.

It is important to note that "equity" is not the same as "equality." Equality suggests that all individuals will be given the same opportunities and access to resources. In contrast, equity takes into account existing disparities between individuals to acknowledge that varying levels of support may be required to achieve similar outcomes. A classic example is that of three individuals watching a baseball game from behind a wooden fence, equipped with multiple, equal-sized boxes between the three of them to stand on [4].

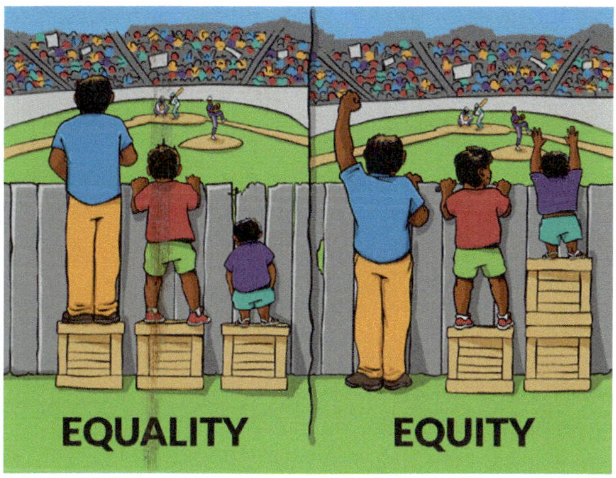

Illustrating Equality vs. Equity (Maguire, 2016).

Illustrating Equality **vs.** *Equity* **[4]**

The one individual, being much taller, does not need any boxes to see over the fence and watch the game. In contrast, the two shorter individuals need 1 and 2 boxes, respectively, to see over the fence. In reality, the allocation of healthcare resources often amounts to a gigantic chasm between high and low socioeconomic classes. The tall individual, the high socioeconomic status (SES) individual in this case, is provided countless boxes, towering over the fence, while the lower SES individuals are provided only one or none at all and are unable to watch the game. In an equal world, each person gets one box. Unfortunately, while the tall and slightly shorter individuals can see over with ease, the shortest individual is still left unable to watch the game. Now, in an equitable world, each individual gets exactly what they need, splitting the boxes so that all individuals are able to finally watch the game. This is the case with justice within healthcare, as we strive to grant individuals comprehensive, timely access to healthcare based on their specific needs. For Ob/Gyn providers, this is ensuring equitable access to reproductive services, such as contraception or prenatal care, as well as reducing existing barriers to accessing care. Such efforts require analysis of the social determinants of health, "the conditions in which people are born, grow, work, live, and age, and the wider set of forces and systems shaping the conditions of daily life," have been found to play a greater role in health status than healthcare services themselves [1].

Now, back to the baseball example: the three friends continue to watch the game, having equitably distributed the boxes to be able to see over the fence. Yet, what we often fail to recognize in this scenario is that there is still a fence separating them from the game and the rest of the fans in attendance. The fence in this case represents the systemic barriers that perpetuate inequity, despite efforts to reduce this chasm in our society and throughout healthcare. Only through addressing the underlying causes of inequity can this fence be torn down, allowing individuals to view the game without the need for support. As healthcare providers, it will be up to you to engage in advocacy efforts to promote social justice and health equity and work toward the elimination of longstanding disparities in maternal and infant health outcomes.

Ethical Dilemmas: Shying Away from "One-Size-Fits-All" Solutions

So how does this play out in clinical practice? Unfortunately, there is no one-size-fits-all approach to ethical decision-making. In a setting of constantly evolving and complex ethical challenges, it will be up to you as Ob/Gyn providers to integrate the foundational ethical principles of autonomy, beneficence, nonmaleficence, and justice into your day-to-day practice. Respect patient autonomy in helping to guide understanding of treatment options to make informed decisions about their care. Prioritize the well-being of the mother and infant through proactive, evidence-based practices that provide the maximum benefit to their health. Strive to minimize harm and maximize safety in all aspects of care. And work to deconstruct systemic barriers and promote equitable access to care for all individuals toward the elimination of longstanding health disparities. As champions of ethical healthcare, Ob/Gyn providers have the ability to shape a better future for reproductive medicine.

Works Cited

1. Centers for Disease Control and Prevention. Social Determinants of Health at CDC. Centers for Disease Control and Prevention. 2022, December 8. https://www.cdc.gov/about/sdoh/index.html
2. Dupras C, Birko S, Affdal A, Haidar H, Lemoine ME, Ravitsky V. Benefits, challenges and ethical principles associated with implementing noninvasive prenatal testing: a Delphi study. CMAJ Open. 2018;6(4):E513–9. https://doi.org/10.9778/cmajo.20180083.

3. Ghi T, Sotiriadis A, Calda P, Da Silva Costa F, Raine-Fenning N, Alfirevic Z, McGillivray G. ISUOG Practice Guidelines: invasive procedures for prenatal diagnosis. Ultrasound Obstet Gynecol. 2016;48:256–68. https://doi.org/10.1002/uog.15945.
4. Maguire A.. Illustrating equality vs. equity. Interaction Institute for Social Change. Interaction Institute for Social Change. 2016. Retrieved May 2024, from https://interactioninstitute.org/illustrating-equality-vs-equity/
5. Primum non nocere. Oxford Reference. Retrieved May. 2024., from https://www.oxfordreference.com/view/10.1093/oi/authority.20110803100345841
6. Uniformed Services University of the Health Sciences. Timeline of landmark events in the evolution of bioethics. Uniformed Services University of the Health Sciences; 2021. https://www.usuhs.edu/sites/default/files/2021-06/TimelineofLandmarkEventsinBioethics.pdf

Chapter 40
Litigation

Robin Perry

After spending over a decade training to provide quality healthcare for women, we feel very comfortable in the world of medicine, with the vocabulary of medicine and the culture of medicine. When we are named in a malpractice suit and experience the litigation process, we are introduced, quite abruptly, to an entirely different world—the world of law and the legal system, which has its own vocabulary and its own culture. The difficulty this poses for obstetrician gynecologists is that, while we already feel vulnerable and stressed by an adverse outcome, we are then immersed in a foreign world with a culture and vocabulary we don't completely understand to determine whether we are guilty or not guilty of malpractice. In this chapter I want to familiarize you with the process of litigation, some of the vocabulary you will encounter while going through the process, and some aspects of the culture of the legal system. I will also make some suggestions as to how you can cope with the stress associated with the process.

Adverse Events

In the chapter on malpractice, we reviewed some aspects of how to approach the adverse event. Not all litigation begins with an adverse event, but many claims do. An adverse event is when a patient injury results from medical intervention, rather than the patient's underlying condition. Not all adverse events lead to lawsuits. However, if there is an adverse event and there is an error, or even a perceived error,

R. Perry (✉)
Division of Maternal-Fetal Medicine, Department of Obstetrics and Gynecology, Cooper Medical School of Rowan University and Cooper University Health Care, Camden, NJ, USA

A. Malik et al. (eds.), *An Obstetrician/Gynecologist's Path*,
https://doi.org/10.1007/978-3-031-87098-9_40

this combination will often lead to a liability claim. Recognize that adverse events can lead to malpractice claims and begin to emotionally and intellectually prepare when the adverse event occurs.

It is important to recognize that an unexpected adverse outcome can be a major trauma for physicians as well as our patients and their families. The adverse event can leave us with feelings of guilt, anger, fear, sadness, and helplessness. We may feel overwhelmed that we have somehow caused the adverse event. We often try to identify a cause and sometimes try to assign responsibility or even blame. When reviewing the adverse event, we should try to avoid being unfairly judgmental of our own competence. We should also avoid being so defensive that we are unable to admit that we may have contributed to the outcome. Learning from these experiences is what makes us excellent. Dealing with the adverse event in an emotionally healthy way is the first step toward coping well with a malpractice claim.

My advice on coping with an adverse event is to first acknowledge the importance of the event. These events are major life-changing experiences. I would recommend talking to others about what happened, taking care when choosing who to speak with regarding the details of the case, and as always, remember your obligations under health insurance portability and accountability act (HIPAA). It is important that we speak openly with our loved ones about our feelings and the impact the event has had on our life. When facing this type of stress, it is important to prioritize self-care, eating healthy foods, getting exercise, and making sure we have time for ourselves to do things we enjoy. Last, it's important to self-monitor our behavior for evidence of serious stress like sleeplessness, increased alcohol consumption, or self-medication. If these issues occur, seeking professional advice around managing the stress becomes essential.

On the practical side, when an adverse event occurs, it is important that we inform our insurance claims carrier. The hospital risk manager should also be notified. Sharing the event with the partners in your practice is also important since they will be managing the patient with you after the event. The importance of detailed, honest documentation cannot be overstated. You should read the entire chart and be familiar with what has been documented by the entire healthcare team. Never alter any medical records, as they are legal documents. If a correction needs to be made, it should be made as an addendum.

When an adverse event occurs, it is important for us to honestly consider what our role is in the event. Sometimes we can be overly critical of our own performance, and other times denial can get in the way of an honest evaluation. Take the time needed to establish some emotional distance from the event and then review the chart with an open mind. If there is concern that the medical record, while accurate, does not reflect the entirety of the circumstances of the adverse event, we can review the concerns with our risk management team. One option to consider is preparing a written narrative of our recollection of the case from beginning to end, as a communication to our attorney, in anticipation of a potential claim. Doing this soon after the event will help to keep the event fresh in your mind. This is especially important since it can take a year or two for a claim to be filed and 3 or 4 years for it to go to trial. All attorney-client communications are privileged.

Malpractice Claims

There are some warning signs that a clinical case may lead to a malpractice claim. Any unexpected negative outcome can lead patients and their families to file a claim. Contact from any attorney who is not retained by the practice may be a sign of a problem. It is best to hold off on providing information to a plaintiff's or potential plaintiff's attorney until you have contacted your liability insurance carrier for advice. Evidence of patient dissatisfaction, like changing physicians or not following advice can also be warning signs that a malpractice claim is being considered.

The Complaint

Litigation (or the process of taking legal action) begins when the patient (now termed the plaintiff or the person bringing the suit to court) files a complaint at the courthouse. A complaint is a legal document containing the allegations. The language used in a malpractice complaint is often inflammatory, using terms like "recklessly, negligently and wantonly." This is an example of the culture differences I mentioned above. Complaints are often written to describe the person who the complaint was filed against (now termed the defendant) and their actions in a negative light. When reading the first complaint that was ever filed against me, I was stunned. I could not imagine that anyone who knew me could describe me or my practice in such terms. I have come to learn that these terms are standard boilerplate for these types of documents. Don't take it personally.

Service of Process

After the complaint is filed, the defendants need to be officially notified. The formal delivery of the summons and complaint is called the "service of process.". We are "served" with a written document notifying us that a complaint has been filed against us, describing the claims that have been made. In some states, the summons is mailed and in others the sheriff's deputy delivers the summons in person. For individuals in states that are served in person, it is advisable to have office personnel who are prepared to remove the deputy from public spaces for the service of process.

Once served with the summons and complaint, we need to inform our insurance carrier, and then we will be assigned an attorney. At this point the adverse event has become a malpractice complaint. Realize that a year or two may have passed since the adverse outcome, before the summons and complaint are received. We may not even remember the patient involved. When we recall the clinical scenario, particularly if it was emotionally traumatic, we may experience a resurgence of the original stress associated with the adverse outcome. In addition to the recurrent stress, we will experience the stress of anticipating going through the litigation process. Having some coping skills at this stage could be very advantageous. First, we want to realize that we are entering into a world that we are not familiar with and that self-preservation is our goal. There are many things that are outside of our control; however, we should take control of that which we can. We can educate ourselves about the litigation process. We can work to achieve comfort and equilibrium in the other areas of our lives. We should do what we can to maintain emotional balance, like avoiding situations that generate anxiety, participating in leisure activities and sports, re-evaluating our time commitments to work and our personal life, taking time for a vacation, and sharing our feelings with trusted individuals. Again, when responding to an adverse event, focus on self-monitoring for concerning behaviors. One of the most important things to remember about the process of litigation is that it is about compensation, not competence.

Pretrial Discovery

The next phase of the litigation process is pretrial discovery. Discovery is the process of gathering facts and opinions from the parties in the case. It is used to better understand who the witnesses are and what they intend to say at trial. Pretrial discovery includes interrogatories and depositions.

Interrogatories

Interrogatories are a series of written questions that we are asked to complete prior to the deposition. We can work with our lawyer on the responses to interrogatories, or they can be completed without an attorney. In my experience, some of these questions can be very vague and nonspecific. It is important to remember to answer just the questions that were asked.

Deposition

A deposition is testimony given under oath in response to questions by the plaintiff's attorney. The deposition has multiple purposes. It forces us to commit to a set of facts, identifies others who may have knowledge about the case, evaluates the defendant (us) to determine what kind of impression we will make on the jury, and elicits testimony that can later be used for impeachment (used against us). The experience of being deposed is quite unique. Depositions occur with you (the defendant) under oath in a setting where a court stenographer is recording everything said.

Alternatively, the deposition could be videotaped. The methodology of a deposition is that the defendant answers only the questions that are asked by the plaintiff's attorney. This often makes us feel like we have been denied the ability to tell our story, which can lead to anxiety and frustration. Depositions place us at the center of attention in a foreign setting. The plaintiff's attorney, however, is in a completely different position. The plaintiff's attorney, in a deposition, feels the same way we feel in a delivery room or operating room, completely comfortable and in their element. The plaintiff's attorney will use multiple techniques to elicit testimony that can later be used for impeachment. The plaintiff's goals at the time of deposition are to lock us into a set of facts, generate impeachable testimony, possibly make us lose control, and get us to agree to things that make the plaintiff's case easier. In my experience, the defendant rarely feels that a deposition was successful, but it is a success when we do not allow the plaintiff's attorney to achieve their goals.

Preparing for a deposition is extremely important. We should prepare for our deposition as we would prepare for an oral board examination: know the patient's chart, prepare by role-playing, and prepare answers to expected difficult questions. There are strategies that can help us have a successful deposition. If possible, have the deposition occur in a familiar location to minimize stress. While we cannot control the plaintiff attorney's questions, we can control the tone and pace of the deposition. Pause and think about the responses to a question when needed. If a question seems inappropriate, look toward the defense attorney and give them time to object. When a question is unclear, ask for clarification. When a break in the proceedings is needed, ask for one. Depositions can take many hours to complete; they are over when the plaintiff's attorney has no more questions. Some cannot be completed in one day. It is entirely reasonable to take a break every two hours or as needed. Some attorneys utilize sarcasm and criticism as a technique in depositions. We should respond to sarcasm and criticism with thoughtful answers delivered calmly. Throughout the deposition, keep calm and do not respond emotionally; we want to be formidable opponents.

Expert Witnesses

After discovery has been completed and the facts have been identified, expert testimony is obtained for both sides. Obtaining an appropriate expert is something you might be asked about. While reputation and renown are important in the selection of an expert, it is also important in trial law for the expert to be persuasive and knowledgeable, to make complex medical information understandable, and it doesn't hurt if they have charisma. The experts for both sides will provide their opinions on the case. When all this information is gathered, the possibility of settling the case is considered.

Settlement

Settling a case can be a double-edged sword. On the one hand, settling means you would not have to go through the trauma of a trial, but on the other hand, you will not have the opportunity to tell your story in open court and have the chance to be found not guilty by a jury. Some malpractice coverage policies give the physician the authority to refuse settlement, and others do not. The decision regarding settlement is multifactorial and complex. Things to analyze can include (1) an objective evaluation of the strengths and weaknesses of the expert testimony, (2) consideration of what exactly the records say, (3) does the plaintiff evoke sympathy, (4) could the jury award exceed your policy limits, (5) how do juries in the geographic area usually behave, (6) what does the claims representative think, and (7) what will the trial cost. The decision regarding settlement should be made based on the merits of the case and not our emotions. Consider how ending the case might contribute to our emotional and financial health. It is not a bad idea to get some objective advice to help sort out the myriad of feelings associated with settlement by reaching out to family, trusted friends, senior colleagues, or perhaps a private attorney.

The Trial

Going to trial has been compared to going to war by some. It requires all our energy and resources. We will play a critical role in our own defense. It's important to acknowledge our feelings prior to trial so that we can project a calm and professional demeanor during the trial. Unplanned delays in the scheduling are common and can be very frustrating. The trial will begin with jury selection. We, as the defendant, can participate in jury selection. Be aware that entering a courtroom for the first time as a defendant and sitting up front at the defendant's table can be a humbling and disturbing experience. I recommend bringing a support person to the courtroom throughout the trial. The trial starts off with opening statements from both sides. Hearing the way the plaintiff's attorney frames events for the jury can be upsetting. Be prepared to hear arguments designed to persuade the jury to decide for the plaintiff. After opening statements, the court will hear testimony from witnesses for the plaintiff and the defense. When giving testimony, be extremely well prepared, address the jury when speaking, use teaching skills to explain responses, maintain composure at all times, and follow the defense attorney's clues. Remember that testimony continues beyond the courtroom. What might be overheard in a restroom by a member of the plaintiff's team can find its way into testimony. After all testimony has been given, both sides have an opportunity to present their closing statement. After closing statements, the jury is instructed on necessary points of law by the judge, and they are released to deliberate. The amount of time that the jury takes to deliberate varies. When the jury has come up with a verdict, our attorney will be informed, and we are called back to court to hear the verdict.

I must be honest and say that even if you win, you feel like you lost. The feeling is not unlike how you feel after your oral board examination. Of course, you are happy to have been found not guilty, but the process itself is somewhat punishing and a bit traumatic. When we lose a trial, there is so much to process. No case goes to trial if there was clear malpractice; we have insurance coverage for those cases, and they are predominantly settled. Losing at trial can feel soul crushing. It is essential to remember that the litigation process is about money, not clinical competence. Juries are made up of people who, when they see the impact of an adverse outcome on the plaintiff, want to try to compensate them. This could cause some jury members to have a very liberal definition of negligence. This is why so many cases are settled. Learn what you can from your experience, and acknowledge that it may take years to fully process what was experienced. After a trial it is particularly important to self-monitor for signs of depression. Keep perspective—over a career we will care for thousands of patients; this is just one, and this one outcome does not define us.

Understanding the litigation process helps to demystify it for the medical professional. While the process is long and complex, understanding the sequence of events and the terminology used can help to diminish stress. To bring perspective to the discussion, consider the following data. According to a 2017 study [1], regarding procedural ObGyn malpractice claims, 59.5% of claims were dropped, withdrawn, or dismissed, while 27.7% were settled. A total of only 8.6% of claims went to trial, with the vast majority, 87.2% of trials, being decided for the defendant and only 12.8% of trials obtaining a verdict for the plaintiff. The litigation process, though daunting, offers us a unique opportunity to refine our practice, strengthen our resolve, deepen our empathy, and grow as professionals.

Reference

1. Glaser LM, Alvi FA, Milad MP. Trends in malpractice claims for obstetric and gynecologic procedures, 2005 through 2014. Am J Obstet Gynecol. 2017;217(3):340.e1–6. https://doi.org/10.1016/j.ajog.2017.05.037.

Further Reading

https://www.acog.org/practice-management/professional-liability

Part IV
Long Term Goals and Planning

Chapter 41
Leaving Your First Job

Ciaran Smolinsky

Job Search

In addition to all that is covered earlier in this book, there are a few extra things to consider when you are ready to leave your first position after residency. When you start looking for a new position, be familiar with your current contract to see what restrictive covenants you are obligated to follow and how that may affect your job search. There may also be consequences for leaving before the conclusion of the initial term; you should be aware of whether you may be required to pay back a portion of a sign-on bonus you received or if you could lose some of the money your employer has contributed to your retirement accounts if there is a vesting schedule. Hopefully your first contract does not require you to be responsible for malpractice insurance tail coverage, but if it does, be prepared to arrange (and pay a lot of money for) this coverage.

Depending on your situation, you may not want it known that you are considering a job transition until you have a new position lined up. It is perfectly reasonable to ask for discretion when submitting applications or talking with recruiters if you do not want your current employer to know you are looking to make a change. But obstetrics and gynecology can be a small community and eventually word could get back to your employer, especially if you are looking locally. Most practices will require references, and if you are not ready to reveal your plans yet, consider using references from residency or other physicians outside your group who have worked with you in a clinical setting. While interviewing, you should be prepared to answer questions about why you are leaving (and have an idea of how to frame it in a positive way).

C. Smolinsky (✉)
Department of Obstetrics and Gynecology, Lankenau Medical Center, Wynnewood, PA, USA

A. Malik et al. (eds.), *An Obstetrician/Gynecologist's Path*,
https://doi.org/10.1007/978-3-031-87098-9_41

Logistics

Once you have decided to leave your first position, you should update your contact information for your various professional accounts (ACOG, ABOG, CAQH, DEA, state medical board, etc.) so you don't lose access when you are no longer an employee (you will likely no longer be able to use your email address with your employer once you leave your position). You will also lose access to patient records. This is particularly important if you have been collecting cases for the ABOG certifying exam. You should make sure you have access to whatever information (in a de-identified, HIPAA compliant manner) you might need to prepare for the exam after you leave. The following is a list of other items you should have copies (or originals) of before you leave your first position:

- Medical license and DEA card
- Record of continuing medical education (CME)/certificates
- ACLS and BLS certifications (check expiration dates)
- OR preference cards
- EMR templates
- Surgical dictation templates
- HIPAA compliant procedure logs
- Malpractice insurance face sheet (and information about tail coverage if applicable)
- PowerPoints or lectures you've given
- Important emails that you wish to keep
- Previous contracts
- Vaccination records, TB tests, etc.

If you will be moving for your next position, you should consider whether you will need to take some time off from your current job to look for housing in your new location or if you might need to have a delay between leaving your first position and starting your second to allow for time to move and get settled in your new home. There may be a lot of time-consuming tasks (updating your driver's license and registration if you move out of state, enrolling children in school or daycare, registering your pets, setting up utilities, etc.) that you might want to complete before starting your new position.

Timing

Transitioning to your second job will take longer than you think. The process of applying for a new position, interviewing, and receiving and comparing offers will probably take you at least 2–3 months. Once you've decided where you'll go next, having your attorney review (and possibly negotiate) your contract can also take weeks to months. Then, when the contract is finalized and signed, the process of credentialing will probably drag on for several more months. Make sure that you are not the hold-up—be proactive about completing whatever paperwork you can (background checks, malpractice applications, insurance forms, obtaining a new state medical license if necessary…) as soon as possible, but be prepared that your start date may eventually get pushed back. This entire process can easily take 6–9 months to complete, and potentially more if you are open-minded about the type of position or geographical area you are considering.

This brings up the delicate matter of when to tell your current employer that you will not be working with them forever. Check your current contract and make sure you understand how to leave. You will need to give notice per whatever time period is required in your contract (90–120 days is common). Some contracts may stipulate *how* notice is to be given and to whom (e.g., written notice, via certified mail, etc.). You should also be aware that some employers may no longer accommodate your requests for CME, vacation, etc., once you have given notice. This is a judgment call, but most advice advocates for giving the minimal notice necessary—you don't want to end up with an unplanned period without pay or benefits if you let them know your plans sooner and they decide they don't need you to stay on beyond the required notice period.

Your Accounts

Make sure you know how to access your accounts (401(k), 403(b), 457(b), Health Savings Account, Flexible Spending Account, etc.) before you leave your first position. This includes knowing your account provider, website, username, and password. You should update your contact information for each account to reflect your personal email address.

You should also be aware of your options for what to do with the money in those accounts when you leave—what you choose can have hefty tax consequences, and if you aren't sure of the best option for you, you may want to consult an advisor. Depending on your specific plan and the amount you've contributed to your account, you may be able to keep your savings in your former employer's plan or you can perform a rollover to a new plan. You should compare investment options and fees between plans. If you receive a distribution from your 401(k) or 403(b) and do not quickly transfer it to a new qualified account (like a 401(k), 403(b), or traditional IRA), you will have to pay taxes and an early withdrawal penalty. If you convert into a Roth IRA you will need to pay taxes on the amount unless your former account was also a Roth. If you will be self-employed or doing locum tenens, look into self-employed retirement plan options such as an individual 401(k) or SEP IRA. And remember, just because you transferred money into an account with your new employer, the money is not necessarily automatically invested; you will need to choose your investments and set up your contributions through your new position.

Your Benefits

You will typically lose your benefits, including health insurance, once you leave your employer. If there is a gap in coverage between the time you leave your first position and when you become eligible for coverage with your new employer, you should consider your options for interim health insurance coverage:

- Joining a spouse's plan: Leaving your job is considered a qualifying life event, and if you have a spouse with an insurance plan through his or her employer, you may be able to join the plan. If your transition occurs outside of the annual open enrollment season, you will need to request a special enrollment period. This is time-sensitive so you should begin this process as soon as you know when you will be losing your benefits.
- Consolidated Omnibus Reconciliation Act (COBRA): Through COBRA, you can continue your coverage with the group health plan sponsored by your first employer after leaving your position. You will typically have 60 days to elect COBRA coverage and can continue coverage for up to 18 months. Your monthly payment for COBRA coverage is likely to be much higher than your premium while employed because your former employer will no longer be subsidizing the cost of the plan for you.
- Obtaining private health insurance: Through the Health Insurance Marketplace, you can compare health insurance plans and pricing. If your job transition occurs outside the open enrollment period, you will usually have a 60-day window to apply for a special enrollment period and select your new coverage.

You should also be aware of any gaps you might have in other benefits such as life insurance and disability insurance if provided by your employer. Even if you begin your new job immediately after leaving your first position, you may not be eligible to participate in some benefits until you have been employed for a certain amount of time.

Take Something with You

Your first position might not have been your perfect forever position, but you definitely got something out of it. Perhaps you got exposure to a new health system with different ways of doing things than your residency institution. Maybe it was just the confidence of managing patients on your own or the ability to handle a busy office schedule. Maybe you collected cases for your boards, met a mentor, or got a better idea of how you want your long-term career to look. You probably had some meaningful patients who will forever impact how you practice medicine. Take what you've learned with you to your new job. Try to be gracious when you are leaving and don't burn bridges on the way out. Most importantly, work well up through the day you leave.

Chapter 42
Learning New Skills

Kathleen Schaeffer

After finishing residency in 2005, I decided to continue working at the Institution where I trained because I enjoyed the challenging patient population and the teamwork mentality that existed in our department. While staying to work at your home institution has definitive advantages, a concern can be the difficulty of bringing new skills to the residents and medical students you will train. To offset this, I decided to take on leadership roles early in my career to provide new challenges and give me something additional to offer in mentoring residents and medical students. Regardless of where you go, learning new skills and challenging yourself can open up new opportunities and make you a more effective physician and teacher. This chapter outlines my own journey in continuously learning new skills, which I offer as an example of how you might find your own path in doing the same.

Early on in my career, I accepted the position of Assistant Residency Program Director. This afforded me the opportunity to work with the program administration. In this role I learned all the technical aspects of running a residency program and was able to implement changes in our simulation sessions and interviewing process. At the APGO/CREOG meetings, I found myself drawn toward sessions that had to do with simulation and prevention of resident attrition. I incorporated concepts from these sessions to enhance the gynecology simulations at my institution. I also initiated a behavior-based interviewing style in our recruitment process to acquire a cohesive group of residents into our small program, as I learned the best step to preventing attrition was careful selection. Introducing behavioral interviewing at that time was relatively new, and implementing the change took several steps. I first had to obtain approval for this new interviewing style from the program director. Upon reviewing this concept and the potential positive impact on our program,

K. Schaeffer (✉)
Department of Obstetrics and Gynecology, Cooper Medical School of Rowan University and Cooper University Health Care, Camden, NJ, USA

A. Malik et al. (eds.), *An Obstetrician/Gynecologist's Path*,
https://doi.org/10.1007/978-3-031-87098-9_42

I was given permission to move forward with this project. Initially, I met resistance from the tenured members of our faculty and had difficulty convincing them that these changes would be a successful endeavor. Introducing a new style meant changing our interviewing process entirely, from application review, format of interview days, and how we would create rank order lists. It would require dedicated faculty to be trained in this interviewing style. This altered the culture of our interviews but created expertise among a small group of faculty members and helped us to learn more about the applicants during the interview process. Each year we reassessed this process and modified things to make the interviewing process stronger, and each year we saw our matched applicants get stronger. This change ultimately helped to obtain the goal of decreasing attrition in the program.

A bit later in my career, I also wanted to expand my skills as a gynecologic surgeon and was fortunate to have a mentor in this area. Those interested in gynecologic surgery will quickly realize there will always be a new technique or equipment to learn. In my case, I wanted to start performing robotic and advanced laparoscopic surgeries, but I had minimal exposure to laparoscopic hysterectomies and complex laparoscopic surgeries in residency. To narrow in on these areas, I needed to seek out training and information on these techniques. I went through the online and animal lab training for robotics and had my mentor proctor the required five cases. I practiced frequently and watched other surgeons both in person and in video recordings. I then started identifying patients who required robotic hysterectomies. One thing I quickly realized is that in learning new skills, there will never be a perfect first patient. You need to be willing to take newly acquired skills and work your way through the difficulties of performing these surgeries. As with acquiring any new skill, it will require additional hours in the OR. It can be helpful to seek out OR block time, connect with equipment representatives, and prepare patients to work through procedures as you are adjusting to the new equipment.

As an attending physician, you will always have opportunities to continue learning. Anyone involved in teaching will have to continuously learn new skills for effective feedback, communication, and information dissemination. Additionally, it is likely that just a few years out of training you will see that what you learned in residency may not continue to be the standard of how you will care for your patients. You will need to decide how much time you want to spend learning these new procedures and treatments; these decisions will ultimately shape your specific practice within OB/GYN. Learning new skills will entail significant time outside your comfort zone, especially if you want to become an expert in that area. It is helpful to seek out mentors at your local institution or through the yearly meetings of national organizations where other physicians are sharing their knowledge. It is important to be confident in yourself even when you are developing new skills and abilities. Ultimately, this ability to learn new things and apply them to multiple facets of your job is what makes practicing within the field of OB/GYN dynamic and exciting.

Chapter 43
Military Surgery

Kristen Knapp and John Chovanes

In the fall of 2019, I was a 4th-year medical student buried deep in an existential crisis about what to do with my life. I was torn not only between specialties—should I pursue surgery, my true passion, or emergency medicine, which boasted an easier lifestyle and shorter training—and also paths in clinical medicine—was it finally time to join the military, or would I be signing my life away?

I'd always planned to join the military at some point, having grown up with mentors, family, and friends in all branches of the armed forces. There are many points in a medical career that a physician can join the military, and I had considered all of them. For those ready to fully immerse in military medicine, there's the highly selective Uniformed Services University of the Health Sciences (USUHS)—the military's medical school. Acceptance into USUHS, which is highly competitive, incurs a 7-year active duty service obligation in the Army, Navy, Air Force, or U.S. Public Health Service after completion of residency. Of note, the Marines do not have a medical force and instead are served by Navy medicine. Students enjoy the benefits of active duty pay, housing allowance, tuition-free medical education, and early exposure and immersion in military life. Unfortunately, with my unconventional academic background and no prior military service, I was not offered an interview.

Thankfully, there are other ways to join the military medical force as a medical student. The Health Professions Scholarship Program (HPSP) is available to any student accepted to a US civilian medical school, through all branches of the military—Army, Navy, and Air Force—as well as the U.S. Public Health Service. When I was accepted to medical school at the University of Virginia, I engaged with recruiters from every branch. The benefits of the HPSP program are the same

K. Knapp (✉) · J. Chovanes
Department of Surgery, Division of Trauma Care, Acute Care Surgery and Surgery Critical Care, Cooper Medical School of Rowan University and Cooper University Health Care, Camden, NJ, USA

A. Malik et al. (eds.), *An Obstetrician/Gynecologist's Path*,
https://doi.org/10.1007/978-3-031-87098-9_43

regardless of the service chosen—scholarship recipients are commissioned as second lieutenants in their branch of choice, which pays all medical tuition and fees, and receive a monthly stipend of over $2500. Depending on the branch, students may also receive a signing bonus and 45 days active duty pay. In return, for each year the scholarship is accepted, students incur a year of active duty commitment. During medical school, students are required to spend 45 days a year in active duty. Between years 1 and 2, required basic officer training fulfills this requirement. For the remaining clinical years, rotations at military hospitals count towards active duty time, and students are paid as such.

Upon graduating from medical school, students may apply to both military and civilian residency programs in most cases. However, their specialty and residency choice can be affected by the needs of the military. In specialties where military need is high (internal medicine, pediatrics, emergency medicine, OB-GYN, and general surgery), it would be extremely unlikely to be denied entry into the specialty of your choice. However, should one desire a less common specialty, such as ENT or ophthalmology, if the military currently had a surplus of physicians in this subspecialty and low predicted future need for this specialty, the student could be pushed into another specialty for which the military had a high need. Similarly, if a student desired to match into a civilian residency, but military residency spots remained unfilled, that student might be denied the opportunity to join the civilian match. In this unusual situation, the student would have the option to either enter a specialty or residency according to their branch's needs or accept a GMO position (Graduate Medical Officer) for a year or more, then re-attempt the match in the future. A GMO provides primary care in their branch of choice and provides an opportunity to support soldiers, sailors, marines, or airmen in operational units.

By the beginning of medical school, I had been accepted for HPSP in the army, navy, and air force. Having no idea what specialty I might find myself attracted to, however, I did not accept my commission for fear of having my specialty choice reassigned or needing to complete multiple GMO tours without a promise of eventual acceptance into my residency of choice. That being said, all my friends from medical school in the Army, Navy, and Air Force HPSP spoke highly of their experiences and are now in specialties and residency programs they love. By the time residency applications rolled around in my fourth year of medical school, I was beginning to feel like maybe I had "missed the boat" as I watched my HPSP classmates navigating military rotations, joining in on enriching field exercises, and reaping all the other benefits HPSP has to offer.

Thankfully, during this time I learned there are yet more ways to join the military as a resident. All branches of the military have a reserve incentive program available to residents in eligible specialties: Army STRAP (Specialized TRaining Assistance Program), Navy TMS (Training in Medical Specialties), and Air Force Reserve Stipend Program all offer a direct route into the military as a reserve officer. All boast a stipend of ~$2500 a month during residency, and most offer loan repayment up to $250,000. Time spent in residency contributes to retirement. In return, the resident accrues 2 years of reserve service commitment for every 1 year the stipend is accepted. Upon graduation from residency, they will enter the civilian workforce but must remain ready to deploy as a reserve physician.

Around the time I began to consider the Army's STRAP program, I was rotating as an M4 in the Cooper University Hospital Emergency Department in Camden, NJ. I found myself torn between applying to emergency medicine, with its comfortable lifestyle and short training time, or surgery—a daunting commitment, but the specialty I had found most fulfilling by far. I chose to rotate at Cooper in an effort to convince myself that emergency medicine was the field for me. However, I found myself distracted—drawn to the trauma bay and ORs—and disinterested in the medical problems I encountered in the ED. I wanted to fix things that were broken, not just temporize. As such, I found myself reading the CV of LTC John Chovanes on the Cooper Department of Surgery website. Dr. Chovanes' background stood out to me as similar to mine, and his career path had taken him to many of the destinations I was considering. Prior to medical school, Dr. Chovanes had been an EMT, flight paramedic, and nurse. He went on to complete both medical school and surgical residency at the Philadelphia College of Osteopathic Medicine and Trauma and Critical Care Fellowship at the University of Pennsylvania. Just as I was considering, he had joined the Army Reserves as a surgical resident almost 20 years earlier. Needless to say, I immediately reached out—desperate for advice from someone who had walked a similar path.

If you've spent any time in the medical profession, you know that getting a response to a cold email from an attending surgeon is nothing short of a miracle. But he did, and several days later I found myself sitting in the "Embassy," the hub for military, diplomatic, and field surgical affairs at Cooper Hospital. I was expecting to meet a jaded and bitter doctor who would tell me, like many others had, to steer clear of the profession. Instead, I was met by an energetic surgeon, passionate about his work both at home and abroad. He regaled me with stories from residency and fellowship and told me about his many tours of duty since joining the reserves in 2001: trauma surgeon with the 325th Combat Support Hospital on Contingency Operating Base Speicher in Tikrit, Iraq, 2007; trauma surgeon and the Deputy Commander of Clinical Services at Forward Operating Base Salerno in Khost, Afghanistan, 2010 and 2012; and trauma surgeon at Camp Manion with the 948th Forward Surgical Team during the Third Battle of Fallujah, 2016. He shared many of the interesting clinical challenges he encountered, such as removing an unexploded rocket-propelled grenade from a U.S. soldier, for which he received the Army Commendation Medal for Meritorious Service.

Furthermore, he explained that rather than hurting his civilian career, his position in the Army had allowed him to build Cooper Hospital's "Military, Diplomatic, and Field Surgical Affairs" department, for which he is the Chief Military Surgeon. The department hosts the Military Civilian Trauma Team Training Program, an embedded group of military physicians, nurses, paramedics, and APPs who work and train together at Cooper to be best prepared for deployment, and also trains hundreds of Special Operations Combat Medics (SOCMs) from the U.S. Army Special Forces and Rangers, Navy SEALs, and Marine Recon, army medics, U.S. State Department medical personnel, and more. He also told me about the unique opportunity to work alongside other surgical specialities, such as ENT and Ob-Gyn physicians. In all his stories, this appealed to me the most—the opportunity to work together with a diverse team in an austere environment, committed to a common goal. For example:

> It was the 3rd Battle of Fallujah, summer of 2016, when ISIS was being purged from the city of Fallujah. I was attached to Forward Surgical Team (FST), now called a Forward Resuscitative Surgical Detachment (FRSD), where I had the opportunity to work with dedicated and varied military medical professionals. A normal FRSD comprises 20 personnel—a mix of trauma surgeons, nurses, CRNAs, medics, and other specialists. It is not unheard of that an OB gyn and ENT or a vascular surgeon could be attached to this miniature surgical unit as well. The Battle of Fallujah (some would say the 3rd Battle of Fallujah, with the first and second occurring in the early 2000s, led by the US military) was now being led by Iraqi Counter Terrorism Forces (CTFs). These brave soldiers were augmented by the US Military's aviation, artillery, and surgical capabilities. THe FRST is at the vanguard of these surgical field capabilities. One day we received multiple casualties from an IED. These casualties suffered a variety of injuries, but one of the most pronounced was a midface fragmentation wound resulting in severe facial hemorrhage. As an experienced civilian trauma surgeon, I would normally have vast resources to call upon in this scenario—in this case specifically, interventional radiology, to gain access to the maxillary and facial arteries. However, in the sand dunes, on the edge of Lake Habbaniyah, none of these luxuries were available (Fig. 43.1).
>
> After the airway was secured, the patient anesthetized, and whole blood resuscitation initiated, I was in a quandary as to determine the best way to staunch the hemorrhage. Fortunately my colleague was an experienced ENT who demonstrated a supra-auricular incision through which we were able to gain access to the transverse facial and maxillary artery allowing us to ligate and pack with a topical hemostatic (Fig. 43.2). This incision, not normally within the armamentarium of the trauma surgeon, was a clear illustration of cross-surgical discipline cooperation. One could easily envision a setting where the OB-gyn similarly has a novel approach to a significant gynecological or pelvic injury.
>
> Unlike US forces, the Iraqi CTFs were limited in the amount of body armor and protective eyewear issued. As a result, the injuries sustained by the counterterrorism forces were a different wounding pattern than US forces typically suffered. During one afternoon, when multiple wounded arrived, we noticed one soldier with a large posterior penetrating wound medial to the scapula. After obtaining airway control, chest tube placement, and initiation

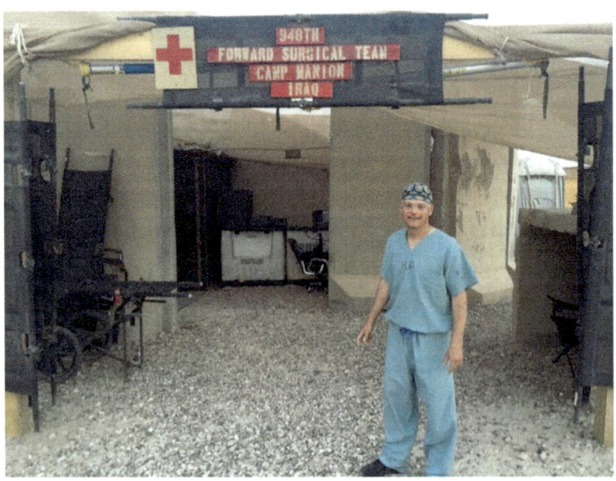

Fig. 43.1 Col Chovanes at the entrance of the 948th FST, Camp Manion, Iraq

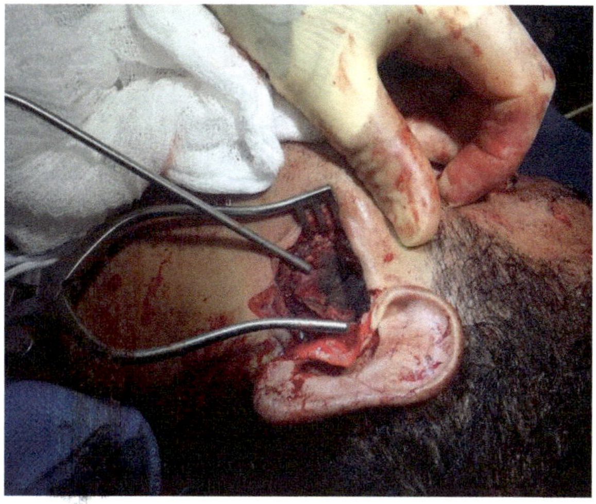

Fig. 43.2 The supraauricular incision demonstrated by Col Chovanes' ENT colleague in a time of need

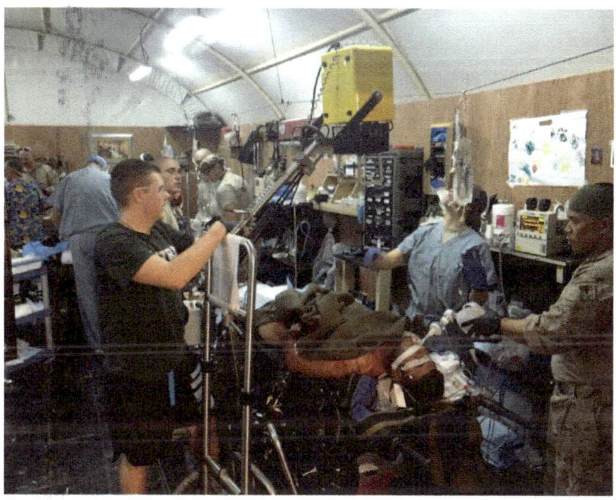

Fig. 43.3 The resuscitation bay at Camp Manion, with multiple casualties being cared for simultaneously after a mass casualty event. In the forefront, a radiograph is in progress, which will identify the fragment of ordinance still present in the Iraqi casualty

of resuscitation, we had the luxury of radiograph (Fig. 43.3). This is not typical FRSD equipment, as imaging is normally limited to ultrasound. The radiograph revealed a large opaque fragment in both the thoracic and abdominal cavities (Fig. 43.4). It was unclear what the fragment was, and concern remained that it could be unexploded ordnance—putting not only the patient, but the entire medical team at risk. Although US Army doctrine for unexploded ordnance in situ is to move the patient to an expectant category and remove them from the treatment facility, this patient was already in the operative suite, as the resuscitation bay and operative suite in the FRSD are in very close proximity to one another.

Because of this, and low probability that this was truly unexploded ordnance, we elected to continue the operation. The patient was positioned for a posteriorlateral thoracotomy, which was successfully completed with the removal of a large jacketed segment of rocket that had entered the patients chest and pressed against his posterior mediastinum and aorta. In this austere setting, a vascular surgeon and a trauma surgeon were able to work in concert to successfully remove the object (Figs. 43.5 and 43.6). The patient was extubated later that

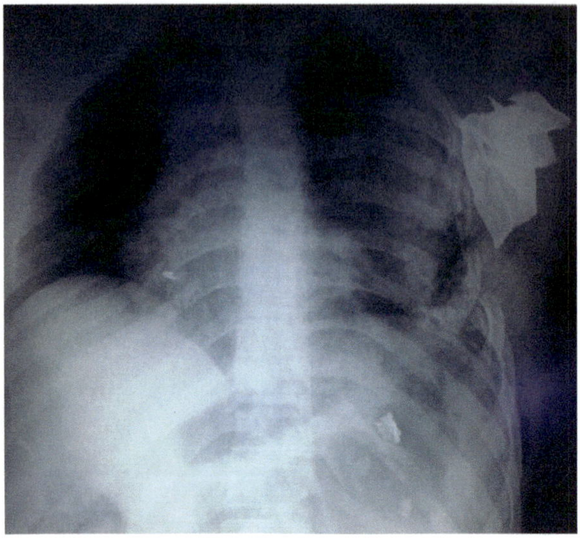

Fig. 43.4 The radiograph demonstrating multiple fragments of ordinance throughout the thoracic and abdominal cavities

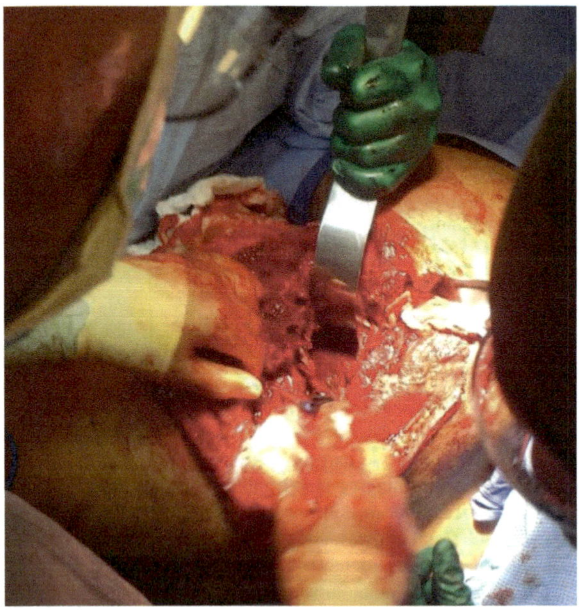

Fig. 43.5 Col Chovanes and his team work together to remove the pieces of ordinance from an Iraqi soldier's chest and abdomen

night and transported in the rear of a humvee back to Baghdad. These cases demonstrate the military surgeon's ability to adapt, improvise, and overcome to result in excellent outcomes.

Needless to say, I left our meeting with the reassurance I needed to charge forward. I matched in general surgery at Cooper Hospital and was commissioned as a captain in the Army Reserves soon after. Now almost 4 years later, I've yet to regret the decision. On the practical side of things, having some extra income during

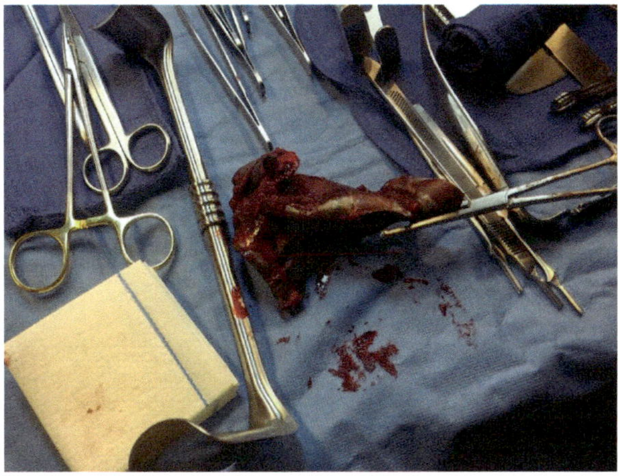

Fig. 43.6 The largest fragment of ordinance after successful removal from the soldiers thoracic cavity

residency has allowed me to provide my family with a much better quality of life during training. More significantly, being in the army has opened up a world of opportunities during training, such as attending military conferences and courses, training medics and police, publishing in military publications, and more—and has never interfered with my residency duties. I've gotten involved with mentoring our medical students in the HPSP program, and I've met incredible teachers, such as Colonel Kirby Gross, who joined the team at Cooper just as my residency began and recently retired from the army at age 70 after over 20 years of service and ten deployments.

Thousands of years ago, the father of medicine, Hippocrates, stated, "He who wishes to be a surgeon should go to war." So many of our medical advances have stemmed from conflict, and the innovation spurred from the human damage war incurs. Being in the military will put me at the forefront of this wave of innovation. Most importantly, however, knowing that I will have a long military commitment ahead of me provides even more motivation to get the most out of my training. Knowing that I'll be responsible for leading a team charged with protecting the lives of our injured soldiers, sailors, marines, and airmen, as well as injured host nationals and even opposition forces, in resource-poor scenarios, often far from additional help and expertise, drives me to soak up every opportunity to advance my knowledge. Our young men and women who put themselves in harm's way to defend our nation deserve the absolute best care medicine has to offer, from the most dedicated team. If this sentiment strikes a chord in your heart as well, consider joining us.

Chapter 44
Pursuing Additional Graduate Degrees or Certifications

Natali Franzblau

Introduction

Life-long learning is a crucial component of medicine. Physicians need to be life-long learners to provide the most up-to-date care to their patients as the advances in medicine continue to evolve. Keeping current with the changes in practice, or becoming a leader in a specific aspect of practice, allows physicians to provide optimal care to patients and is a worthwhile pursuit. Additionally, during their career, some physicians may wonder about expanding their work purview beyond individual patient care and take the lead in something that they are passionate about. Pursuing additional education can provide a broader perspective through interacting with people with similar interests who are coming from different places.

About 10 years into being in practice, I decided to go back to school to get a master's in business administration (MBA). I did a 24-month intensive program that provided me with an education that would allow me to move beyond my role at the time. When I chose that particular program, I had definitive reasons for why I wanted and needed to pursue this additional degree. While I do not regret having done the program, I would give my younger self some food for thought related to pursuing additional degrees or certifications. The information that is included in this chapter is some of what I considered in making the decision to pursue my MBA and some of what I hadn't even thought about but perhaps should have.

I would recommend talking to many mentors and colleagues as you consider whether or not to pursue additional education, and if so, what type of education will be best. These conversations should be with those who you currently work with, those who you have worked with in the past, and also people who know you well

N. Franzblau (✉)
Department of Obstetrics and Gynecology, Cooper Medical School of Rowan University and Cooper University Health Care, Camden, NJ, USA

A. Malik et al. (eds.), *An Obstetrician/Gynecologist's Path*,
https://doi.org/10.1007/978-3-031-87098-9_44

but don't work with you. Consider talking to people who are in positions you may want to pursue in the future to learn what those roles are really like on the inside, not just what they look like from the outside.

Possible Programs

There are a wide variety of degree and certificate programs in which a physician can enroll to develop a deeper and wider knowledge base. One option is always to do a fellowship in a subspecialty, either within the specialty of OB/GYN or related to OB/GYN like addiction medicine, palliative care, or clinical informatics. If you think this would be interesting, it is important to make sure the program will accept your OB/GYN training as a prerequisite.

Common graduate degrees for physicians include the MBA, the master's in public health (MPH), or the master's in health administration or medical management (MHA/MMM). An MBA provides the knowledge and skills to succeed in management in many different industries, whereas the MHA and the MMM are specifically focused on the healthcare industry. There are some MBA programs that provide a focus on healthcare through coursework specific to healthcare. The MMM programs are predominantly targeted to physicians. These master's programs can vary in length from 12 to 24 months or longer, depending on the specific program and how it is structured (full-time or part-time). There are also programs that are titled executive programs. These programs are geared to individuals who are working full time, so they are typically offered on weekends or evenings. There are other master's programs that appeal to physicians, including the fields of ethics, education, or research. Programs vary significantly in terms of the amount of time that is done in person and remotely, either synchronously or asynchronously.

There are also many certificate and non-degree programs that can provide physicians with knowledge and skills to advance or modify their careers in other arenas. There are certifications related to patient safety and quality, like Certified Professional in Patient Safety (CPPS), Certified Professional in Healthcare Quality (CPHQ), and Six Sigma. These certifications can provide the physician with the knowledge and skills to advance patient safety and quality in their work environment. There are also certificate programs in many other areas related to healthcare, including informatics, innovation, and leadership.

This additional training can provide you with an education and expertise that you can use to advance or enhance your personal knowledge and skills to apply in either your current position or a new position. There are many programs available, depending on the motivation and desire.

Motivations

The first question to ask yourself is: Why do I want to pursue this degree or certification? Additional questions include: What will I do with this education after I complete it? What is the right degree for me? Where do I see myself in 5 years, 10 years? There are several common motivations for pursuing additional education. There may be more than one reason that is driving you to think about this path.

One motivation is personal growth and enrichment. Working toward a new degree or certificate will expand your knowledge and skills, giving you a broader view of how your current work may fit into a larger picture. It can allow you to better understand what those around you are doing and better communicate with other colleagues. Similarly, there may be a specific area where you know that you can make a difference but need more formal knowledge and skills to embark on your path. A parallel motivator may be that you are already involved in education or leadership, and you think that pursuing specialized training will provide you with needed knowledge and credentials that are required to do your job better.

Some may find that their medical school or residency education did not provide enough in-depth education in a particular area that is important to their current position.

Some may be motivated to pursue these additional programs to achieve career advancement into leadership positions. Additional education may help open doors more easily than would otherwise happen.

Another motivator may be that you are thinking about pivoting your career in another direction but don't want to lose the benefit of your investment of time and training thus far. In this case, you may want to find a way to capitalize on the education and training that you have already undertaken but use it in a new and different way.

It is helpful to identify why you are contemplating this step in your career. It is also important to consider how you will feel if your new educational path doesn't change where you are in your career, or how you will feel if you make changes but find them less satisfying than you anticipated. There are many personal and professional factors and expectations to take into account before you commit to a new path.

Considerations

An additional degree or certification will entail significant time commitment. The demands of clinical practice should not be underestimated, nor should the demands of an additional degree program. When you are doing your clinical work, you need to be able to focus on your patients, and when doing classwork or homework, you need to not be distracted by your clinical work. You need to figure out how to maintain focus on each area at the appropriate times, avoiding distraction to optimize your efficiency. Developing effective time management strategies will be crucial for your success in both your clinical practice and your educational endeavor.

Pursuing a new educational program will require balancing and rebalancing your work life, personal life, and school life. It is important to consider how long the program is, how much class time there is, and how much homework and group project work will be expected. The longer the program, the more frequently you will need to engage in this rebalancing. It is crucial to discuss this new endeavor with the stakeholders in your personal life and in your work life prior to making this commitment. The stakeholders in your work life will include your co-workers and supervisors. It is likely that pursuing additional education will impact your work schedule, and you will need their cooperation in making any adjustments to your work schedule that may be necessary in your endeavor. As important as commitment from those at work is the commitment of those in your personal life. The important people in your personal life, such as a significant other, spouse, or children, will be affected by this new commitment and should be supportive of this undertaking and be willing to accept the impact it may have on them for the duration of the program. Most of those people who are regular parts of your life will be impacted by your pursuit. The amount of this sacrifice will depend on the length and rigor of the program you choose to pursue. Also, it is important to consider your own wellness. While it might seem that you can focus on work and school for the duration of the program, you must schedule time for your own renewal and relaxation as well.

It is important to consider the financial investment that will be necessary to pursue this additional education. If pursuing a degree, there will be tuition. This tuition can vary greatly, depending on the institution, the type of program, and the length of the program. As you balance the reasons for pursuing the degree and the expectations of what you hope to achieve with the degree, it is important to consider the financial cost as part of your equation. Certificate programs often have lower costs for course work. There is often an additional cost for required exams. There may also be additional periodic expenses for recertification exams in some cases. If programs take place at some distance from your home, there may be travel expenses to consider. Additional thoughts: might there be scholarships, employer tuition reimbursement programs, or employer support for tuition if the program you want to pursue aligns with their mission?

Another aspect to consider when looking at programs is the flexibility of the program. When and how is the work done? Does the program require any in-person time, and are there specific deadlines for work and exams that need to be met? Will you be working with other people so that you will need to coordinate multiple schedules to complete the course work? Is this a program that you do on your own time and at your own pace, without having to consider fellow students in completing the program?

Additional Suggestions

If you decide to pursue a degree or certification program, make sure to network with the people who are teaching in the programs as well as your fellow students. These people can provide new ideas and innovations for you to bring back to your practice or health system. They can provide collaboration for projects and can contribute to future job opportunities.

As you are pursuing this education and after you complete it, be sure to maintain these relationships. Also get involved in professional organizations and attend conferences related to your new field of study. Once you have chosen to further your education, get the most out of your investment by maintaining relationships, building new ones, and keeping up with changes in your new field.

Conclusion

In considering the pursuit of a master's degree or certification, consider why you are doing it and what you will do with the additional skills, knowledge, and relationships you gain. Also weigh the positives and negatives of the endeavor, both during the time you are doing it and when you are finished. Include your stakeholders in the decision-making process, and if you decide to move forward with a program, take full advantage of it.

Chapter 45
Transitioning to Education

Jocelyn Mitchell-Williams

Introduction

Medical educators play a critical role in shaping the future of healthcare through leadership, research, innovation, and implementation of curriculum for the next generation of healthcare professionals. The responsibilities of educators encompass a wide range of tasks aimed at providing high-quality education to a variety of learners, including medical students, residents, fellows, junior colleagues, and other healthcare professionals. The field of medicine, including obstetrics and gynecology, continues to evolve with new technologies, procedures, and practice guidelines. Clinicians that are invested in staying up to date with these advances and dedicated to the dissemination of that knowledge are vital to the improvement of healthcare and women's health. Most of us have memories of at least one special educator that helped us to learn key concepts or skills during medical school or residency training. Others have had mentors who helped them design research protocols, prepare for presentations at conferences, or write manuscripts for publication. The intent of this chapter is to provide information on the different pathways to the many roles of a medical educator and how to prepare for them throughout your career.

J. Mitchell-Williams (✉)
Department of Obstetrics and Gynecology, Cooper Medical School of Rowan University and Cooper University Health Care, Camden, NJ, USA

A. Malik et al. (eds.), *An Obstetrician/Gynecologist's Path*,
https://doi.org/10.1007/978-3-031-87098-9_45

Understanding the Role of Educator

Many imagine that teaching is easy or easier than clinical practice, but it is an art that requires additional knowledge and skill, as well as dedication and commitment to do it effectively. A successful medical educator is able to combine their expertise in their medical field with their passion for teaching and mentoring. If you are employed at an academic medical center, there is likely the expectation that teaching is a part of your job. There is also likely the expectation for scholarly work, which can come in the form of medical education. People seeking employment at academic institutions are often aware of this in advance and have the interest and drive to be involved in medical education.

As a new hire at the start of your career, teaching or educational opportunities may not always be an area of interest. You may be asked to give a lecture on a topic that was taught by a departing faculty member or where there is a gap in the content. Nevertheless, it can be an opportunity to hone your teaching skills, advance your knowledge, and make your interest in education known to the institution. You may also be given the chance to moderate small group discussions or teach in standardized patient settings. These are also great opportunities to get involved in education and will eventually lead to more teaching roles.

In addition, you will be expected to participate in teaching in the clinical setting. This may feel more comfortable for you based on your own experience in residency or as a student. Educators can use these times as opportunities to teach about their field. In OB/GYN, you can teach about reproductive health, gynecological conditions, pregnancy, and childbirth while also role modeling effective communication and professionalism. Hands-on teaching of skills through surgical cases or office procedures are valuable and engaging ways to teach as well. Some educators find that they are better at teaching in the clinical setting versus the classroom. Both are extremely valuable and have an impact on educating future physicians.

As a medical educator, you also have the option to be involved in medical education beyond didactics and clinical teaching. There are opportunities to get involved with curriculum development, assessment, mentorship, educational research, and professional development. These can all be considered educational scholarship. There are education committees that are part of the infrastructure of medical schools and residency programs that play key roles in the educational experience of the students or trainees. Before embarking on these activities, it is important for you to understand the responsibilities and requirements of these roles.

Why Do Physicians Transition to Medical Education?

Transitioning from clinical medicine to medical education can be a rewarding experience. People make this transition for many different reasons [1]. Some have a strong passion for teaching and feel it is their calling. We have all met at least one of these individuals along our path. They are like the Pied Piper of medicine with a line of medical students following behind them, imparting medical knowledge that is rapidly absorbed by their eager learners. While not all faculty members think of teaching as their calling, they still gain a strong sense of personal fulfillment that also draws them to education. Student curiosity can be inspiring and exciting. It can also be a motivation to keep you on your toes and up to date with current research, practices, and procedures. There is something very meaningful about contributing to the development of future doctors and having an impact on their careers. Some may leave a legacy through their teaching and mentorship.

Some clinicians may decide to leave or cut back from clinical practice for a change of pace or new experience. Medical education can offer a slower pace and different focus than the often fast-paced, demanding life of clinical practice. It can allow for exploration of a new or modified career that can alleviate some of the stress associated with patient care. It should not, however, be thought of as a way to escape physician burnout. While teaching can offer a good work-life balance through more predictable or flexible hours, it still requires commitment, knowledge, and preparation.

Finally, there are individuals who transition to medical education to advance their careers either through academic promotion, leadership, or research opportunities. Whether advancing in the field of obstetrics and gynecology or more globally in academics and medical education, educators will need to be engaged and stay updated on the latest developments in their field, teaching pedagogy, and accreditation standards. While this can seem daunting, it can be both intellectually stimulating and rewarding.

Making the Transition

As you consider a shift to focus on medical education, identify your personal motivation for doing so. Assess your skills and interests. Know your strengths so that you can identify the aspects of medical education that you might be best suited for or that might appeal to you. Take into consideration your communication skills, teaching style, and your passions. If you feel you have limited teaching experiences, seek out additional opportunities to build your portfolio. This might include serving as an advisor for the student OB/GYN interest group, mentoring a resident, leading a workshop, being a guest speaker or panelist at the medical school, taking a course, or obtaining an advanced degree in medical education.

In addition to exploring and connecting with educators at your local institution, it can also be helpful to network with other educators regionally or nationally. Attending national meetings for your professional organizations can be extremely helpful. Attend an American College of Obstetrics and Gynecology (ACOG) or Council of Residency Education in Obstetrics and Gynecology (CREOG)/ Association of Professors of Gynecology and Obstetrics (APGO) conference and talk to the presenters of educational topics of interest to you. Ask them about their career trajectory and for suggestions of helpful resources. These types of interactions may help you identify individuals who may be willing to mentor you through the process. They may provide valuable insights into the field and even provide leads on job opportunities. The Learn, Serve, Lead Annual Meeting held by the Association of American Medical Colleges (AAMC) may be more suited for those wishing to transition to or learn more about undergraduate medical education and the numerous roles at the medical school level. Volunteering to serve on any of these organizations' committees can also be a great way to meet people and learn about medical education.

If you are just finishing residency and know that you want to be involved in education, make that clear during the interview process and try to negotiate a percentage of your full-time effort (FTE) for teaching in your contract. Of course, you do need to hone your clinical skills as you begin practice, but a 0.10 FTE or even 0.2 FTE for education is not an unreasonable request, especially if you have demonstrated strong teaching skills and involvement during your residency training. Many medical schools will provide clinical instructor appointments to chief residents, so consider pursuing this while still in residency to gain experience and practice your teaching skills. Be sure to express your desire to teach to your supervisor so that you are kept in mind when opportunities arise. Say yes to opportunities—schools and residency programs will always need volunteers for teaching or committees! If you are returning to your former medical school-affiliated hospital for employment, you may be well suited to take on a given teaching role because you are familiar with the curriculum and format. You can use that to your advantage during the hiring process.

Becoming a successful medical educator requires a set of distinct skills and qualities and a commitment to learning and improving. Having a strong foundation in clinical practice is the first step to being a great educator and will provide you with the knowledge and experience to effectively teach students. Strong written and oral communication skills are needed to help convey complex medical concepts to students from various backgrounds and levels of understanding. Equally important is understanding and considering different learning styles, which can help facilitate the engagement of students and the creation of a positive learning environment. Medical educators also need to be adaptable. Healthcare is constantly changing and advancing, and we must be open to new teaching pedagogies, technology, and ideas.

As you progress in medical education, you should develop teaching strategies that allow for students with different learning styles to be successful. This will help lead to more effective teaching and positive evaluations of your teaching. Learning to incorporate technology and innovation into teaching can also be helpful. Virtual reality and simulation are becoming increasingly more popular in educating medical students and residents. Soon artificial intelligence will likely play a role. Having skills in these areas or other new innovations may give you an opportunity to create a niche for yourself at your institution.

It is important to understand the academic and institutional expectations for becoming an educator and progressing academically [2]. You should inquire about this during your job interview, query current faculty members, and review the faculty handbook for additional information. Requirements may vary significantly across institutions, but academic promotion will likely take into consideration your teaching effort, learner evaluations, and service to the institution. Engaging in scholarly activity such as research, presenting at conferences, and publishing may also be expected to demonstrate advancement of medical knowledge and education [2].

OB/GYN faculty generally work with medical students during the clinical phase of their education, providing lectures and bedside training during the third-year clerkship and fourth-year sub-internships. In addition to teaching, for faculty that are heavily involved in teaching efforts, there may be an opportunity to serve as the director for the clerkship or sub-internship. These positions require significant protected administrative time. Individuals in these types of roles need strong communication and organization skills. They must be able to coordinate lecture and clinical rotation schedules, provide student feedback, and gather meaningful assessment data from their colleagues. Clerkship directors will need to be sure that the curriculum meets the needs of medical students and aligns with the objectives of the institution and accrediting bodies. Students need to be provided with feedback that is constructive and helps them improve. Clerkship directors help develop assessment tools that are fair and comprehensive so that a student's clinical skills, knowledge, and professionalism can be evaluated fairly. One of the most rewarding aspects of serving as a clerkship director is getting to offer mentorship and guidance to medical students who are interested in pursuing careers in OB/GYN [3]. You also get to collaborate with other health professionals, such as nurses, midwives, and other physicians, to provide students with a comprehensive understanding of women's health.

Outside of the OB/GYN curriculum, faculty may also have educational opportunities to serve as committee members, course directors, small group facilitators, academic counselors, career advisors, and administrative deans at the undergraduate medical level. There is often a notification that goes out before the start of the academic year, alerting faculty to open committee seats and faculty teaching positions. These positions are often filled by people who have demonstrated a commitment to educational programming and have some experience. These opportunities may require endorsement from your department chairperson, and committee positions may require election from the faculty body or appointment by the dean.

Finding the Right Balance

It may take time to figure out what the right balance of clinical and teaching time is for you. For example, if you plan to continue operating throughout your career, you need to be sure to have sufficient clinical time to maintain your skills. If you want to be a clerkship director, you need to be willing to spend 40–50% of your effort on the education side. Shifting from clinical to educational activities during the same workday can be challenging, especially if the activities are in different buildings or, worse yet, different towns. If possible, avoid didactic teaching on days when you are in the operating room or have heavy patient schedules to minimize the risk of being late or absent from your teaching responsibilities. Investigate the time commitment for any committees you are considering joining to ensure that you can carve out the time on your schedule. Many committees meet during the workday, which may not align with your clinical schedule. Others may meet in the early morning or early evening to account for clinical scheduling. You may need to take this into account if you have personal or family obligations that would prohibit your participation. You will also want to consider the financial impact of incorporating teaching into your career. The remuneration for teaching at the undergraduate medical level may be lower than for clinical effort, especially if you are on a Relative Value Unit (RVU)-based salary model. Despite this, for most people, the satisfaction and lifestyle are worth it.

Conclusion

Being a medical educator can be an extremely rewarding and meaningful part of your medical career. It is another area to focus your knowledge and skills and to improve and develop over your career. There are multiple ways to get involved in medical education, and when you start out, you should explore as many as you can. As you gain experience, you can then focus on a specific area in medical education. Medical educators play a critical role in teaching and mentoring students and trainees, ensuring that the next generation of physicians provide exceptional care to patients and continue to advance healthcare.

References

1. Bartle E, Thistlethwaite J. Becoming a medical educator: motivation, socialisation and navigation. BMC Med Educ. 2014;14:110. https://doi.org/10.1186/1472-6920-14-110.
2. Rushing GD, Mokadam NA. Faculty development: using education for career advancement. Thorac Surg Clin. 2019;29(3):321–8. https://doi.org/10.1016/j.thorsurg.2019.03.009. Epub 2019 May 17. PMID: 31235301.
3. Sims SM, Cox SM, Bhargava R, Everett EN, Fleming A, Graziano S, Morgan HK, Baecher-Lind L, Royce C, Sonn TS, Sutton JM, Morosky CM. Clerkship director confidence in medical student career advising in obstetrics and gynecology. AJOG Glob Rep. 2023;3(2):100187. https://doi.org/10.1016/j.xagr.2023.100187. PMID: 37064782; PMCID: PMC10090429.

Chapter 46
Global Health Career in OB/GYN

Anna Pancheshnikov

Being involved in Global Health (GH) initiatives and/or Global Health Education (GHEd) can be a greatly rewarding and fulfilling endeavor. Consider a definition of GH: "an area for study, research, and practice that places a priority on improving health and achieving equity in health for all people worldwide," [1] and we begin to understand why. After all, most of us enter medicine with this exact goal and priority in mind—to improve the health of all people and to achieve health equity. As we spend years in hierarchical training institutions, deal with unhappy patients, worry about legal action, and are consumed by documentation, emails, and meetings, we ask ourselves, how and why did I end up here? Throughout my training and now early career, I have felt that concentrating on GH/GHEd helped me refocus away from these distractions by clarifying and bringing into focus my original intentions of choosing a career in medicine.

Global Health for Beginners: Where Do I Start?

1. Explore Your "Why"

My path in GH began early on—interpreting for my family at clinics and hospitals as a young child of immigrants and then myself going through another immigration as a teenager. My interest and passion in immigrant and GH work was solidified through overcoming personal and family challenges. So where do you begin your GH journey? With the rise in popularity and exponential growth of GH/GHEd in

A. Pancheshnikov (✉)
Division of Urogynecology, Department of Obstetrics and Gynecology, Cooper Medical School of Rowan University and Cooper University Health Care, Camden, NJ, USA

A. Malik et al. (eds.), *An Obstetrician/Gynecologist's Path*,
https://doi.org/10.1007/978-3-031-87098-9_46

universities, medical schools, and hospitals all over the world [2], and with the broad definition of GH, you can begin anywhere and anytime. I believe the first step is to figure out your "why."

The world of GH can be challenging and frustrating. You may choose your training programs carefully based on the reputation of their GH resources, only to learn you cannot participate in these opportunities, and even if you are so lucky, you must use your already limited "free" or vacation time to engage in GH. You may invest time and energy in GH endeavors; meanwhile, your focus on learning "how to be a good resident" and studying for exams may be questioned by your leaders and colleagues. You may volunteer many hours to careful planning and organizing GH endeavors, only to encounter impediments, surprises, and perceived failures. Thus, taking the time to explore your "why" is the key to gaining the confidence to begin your GH journey and to keep your GH focus despite *seemingly* conflicting responsibilities and obstacles.

2. *Find Your Niche*

Somewhat less intangibly, the next step would be to find your niche and get comfortable there, at least for a while. When I was still an undergraduate student, with my eye firmly on medical school and a GH career, I became interested in prevention of vertical HIV transmission efforts. This was a natural transition from high school volunteering in a local AIDS non-profit and syringe exchange program. I devoured literature on the topic and spoke widely and loudly about this budding interest to anyone who would listen (and many who wouldn't). A few months later, I connected with a physician leader in Puerto Rico (PR) who was interested in mentoring me. A few months more, and I was collaborating with him on a pilot project through a university grant. For my study abroad experience, I applied for a Brazilian public health program, gaining priceless experience within the world of HIV in another country, and learning another language along the way. A few years more, and I was conducting a yearlong vertical transmission study in the Dominican Republic (DR) through the Fulbright Research Fellowship. With the significant uncertainty imbued in medicine in general and GH in particular, having my niche, both in topic and region of the world, provided me with comfort and security. Gaining experience in this niche allowed me to apply for and (sometimes) get accepted to various fellowships, scholarships, and opportunities.

Of course, each GH beginning may look slightly different: it may start when you are a high-school volunteer or an experienced attending physician; it may be sparked by a chance opportunity or it may be the fruit of careful and intentional pursuit; it may be related to a topic you are already passionate about or a country you are from, or it may be relevant to your chosen profession or the community where you work. Whatever may be the beginning of your GH spark, cherish and cultivate it, as it will be the backbone from which you will eventually expand and diversify.

Fueling the GH Momentum

3. Plan for Everything, Accept the Unexpected, and Shift When Necessary

During my medical studies and while I continued to be involved in vertical transmission research, I quickly realized my passion lay in women's health and not in the world of infectious disease. As I started OB/GYN residency, I realized even quicker still that I was falling in love with gynecologic surgery rather than the obstetrics sphere. So, what do I do now? After more than a decade in the world of vertical transmission, I found myself at a crossroads: How do I continue to invest in my GH career while transferring my focus from an obstetrics niche to a career in complex gynecologic surgery? After a decade of careful planning, I had to embrace a moment of uncomfortable uncertainty. As OB/GYN trainees, uncertainty is not a new concept for us. We deal with it daily in the delivery room, operating room, and on the wards. In this demanding, straining, destabilizing yet exciting field, we use our previous knowledge, experience, and evidence to guide us in challenging situations. You will eventually be able to do a cesarean section in record speed at your 24th hour of being awake. You will also be able to use your already established GH skills and networks to rethink your future in the field if and when necessary.

And so, between hysteroscopies, I was asked by one of my attendings about my GH involvement and whether there would be any interest in urinary incontinence (UI) teaching and service in the DR. Soon after, through my OB/GYN contacts in the country, we were able to arrange UI teaching in a Dominican maternity hospital. The next year we were able to arrange a few patient evaluations and sling surgeries and follow-ups. Throughout the rest of my residency time and with the close partnership of local and international leaders, I was able to invest and grow a project that would eventually become known as Urogynecology Global Health Initiative (UGHI): a project focused on the development of urogynecologic education, training, and service in the DR. The intensive, extraordinarily detailed planning and organization required to coordinate an international surgical collaboration was only surpassed by the unrelenting, unforeseen shifts necessary to maintain the program alive. And then…a global pandemic to boot!

4. Re-focus on Ethics and Sustainability

GH and GHEd endeavors have long raised criticisms and concerns about potentially limited impact; inappropriate allocation of already scarce resources; unbalanced relationships between high- and low-resource partners; questionable quality and efficacy of medical care provided by trainees and faculty unfamiliar with local health needs, culture, and systems; and fundamental ethical questions about patient consent, privacy, and autonomy in low-resource settings [3, 4]. As you struggle with many of these questions, you can lean on previously developed ethical guidelines such as The Working Group on Ethics Guidelines for Global Health Training (WEIGHT), a set of best practices for GH training developed by an international and multidisciplinary group of GH and ethics experts [4]. Additionally, as you participate and eventually lead GHEd efforts, you may find the paucity of standardization in the field to be alarming. The Consortium of Universities for Global Health (CUGH) was formed to define, standardize, and promote the discipline of GH, and within it, the CUGH GH Competency Subcommittee created interprofessional GH competencies to help us set assessable standards of knowledge and performance and assist in GH curriculum development and evaluation [5]. I suggest you familiarize yourself with both the criticisms of the GH/GHEd field as well as the available guidelines and best practices to address these.

As COVID-19 changed the world as we know it, it forced many GH/GHEd leaders to reimagine the field by refocusing on local issues (glocal health focus), collaborating with community organizations, and exploring virtual education technologies and other innovative approaches [6]. At the time I was starting my Urogynecology fellowship training and trying to decide how and if to continue with UGHI—a project focusing on elective procedures to correct pathologies that affect women's quality of life while a global pandemic was ravaging whole communities. I decided to use UGHI's momentum and the unique uptake of virtual education technologies mobilized by the pandemic to shift the focus of the initiative to longitudinal Urogynecologic education and training. The result was a creation of a year-long basic Urogynecologic curriculum in Spanish geared towards OB/GYN and Urology trainees and physicians in Latin America and the Caribbean with monthly virtual lectures, bi-monthly virtual journal club discussions, and quarterly hybrid procedural simulation training with pelvic models. As COVID-19 restrictions slowly lifted, we were able to restart in-person clinical and surgical training, but now with a sharp focus on capacity strengthening and local expert involvement.

By continually focusing on education and training, incorporating web-based technologic innovations, and engaging with local experts and organizations, we continually strive to improve this GH initiative's sustainability efforts and focus on ethical and inclusive practice.

Global Health for the Advanced

5. *Negotiate Your GH Career*

You are now a GH leader! You have found your passion in women's GH, carefully maintained it despite all obstacles, and have somehow survived training while keeping the GH flame burning. You can now sigh with relief as you finally settle into the perfect OB/GYN GH career, right? In fact, as you start the search for your first attending job, the opportunities to significantly incorporate GH into your career may seem grim. You may be promised 10% effort for GH work, only to discover your "protected time" is that same half-a-day-a-week administrative time everyone else uses for documentation and patient messages. You may be encouraged to connect with already established GH initiatives in the institution, using your PTO time, of course. You may even be afraid to speak about your GH interests, let alone GH career plans, because who would want to hire someone who may be "less productive" or away for longer periods of time?

After receiving some contradictory advice about the prospect of incorporating GH/GHEd into my future career, I decided to at least try to have it all: join a team where I could grow as a Urogynecologist, have strong mentorship and support, teach, and continue to be involved in academics, while also growing and focusing on a GH/GHEd career. Some may call this luck, being at the right place/right time, others may say it was persistence and flexibility, but I was able to find this near-perfect opportunity. In my current (and first!) attending position, I was recruited not only as a junior attending Urogynecologist with a GH Urogynecology initiative but also as the director and founder of a new center for GH and GHEd. When speaking to the dean of the medical school, I recognized the unique opportunity of merging my interests and strengths with a great need and interest in centralizing and formalizing GHEd at the institution. Importantly, I had the strong support of the dean and an experienced and well-respected division leader and the experience, vision, energy, and preparation to inspire confidence.

6. *There Is More Than One GH Path*

This is a serious understatement. From being involved in a GH project once a year to founding and leading a major GH initiative; from participating in a GH fellowship to conducting GH research; from founding a GH center to mentoring individual trainees; from negotiating protected time in your contract to using your personal time as possible; from establishing international collaborations to leading global health efforts with local community organizations—there are countless meaningful ways to incorporate GH into your OB/GYN training and career. The path may be arduous, unpredictable, and tortuous, but often fulfilling, hopeful, and interesting.

To summarize:

1. Figure out your "why" in GH—your incentives and motivations.
2. Find your niche in a topic and/or region of the world and gain substantial experience and expertise in it.
3. Fuel your GH momentum:
   (a) Plan everything, be exceptionally organized, and diligent.
   (b) Accept the many unexpected twists and turns in your path.
   (c) Shift as needed; be flexible, humble, and patient.

4. Focus on GH ethics and sustainability:
   (a) Familiarize yourself with GH ethical concerns and the available guidelines and best practices to deal with them.
5. Negotiate your GH career:
   (a) Be vocal about your GH experience and vision.
   (b) Find leaders who believe in you and understand the importance of GH/GHEd.
   (c) Showcase what YOU can offer your institution through GH.
6. Remember there are countless ways to incorporate GH into your OB/GYN training and career.

References

1. Koplan JP, Bond TC, Merson MH, et al. Towards a common definition of global health. Lancet. 2009;373(9679):1993–5. https://doi.org/10.1016/S0140-6736(09)60332-9.
2. Cox JT, Kironji AG, Edwardson J, et al. Global health career interest among medical and nursing students: survey and analysis. Ann Glob Health. 2017;83(3–4):588–95. https://doi.org/10.1016/j.aogh.2017.07.002.
3. Crump JA, Sugarman J. Ethical considerations for short-term experiences by trainees in global health. JAMA. 2008;300(12):1456–8. https://doi.org/10.1001/jama.300.12.1456.
4. Crump JA, Sugarman J, Working Group on Ethics Guidelines for Global Health Training (WEIGHT). Ethics and best practice guidelines for training experiences in global health. Am J Trop Med Hyg. 2010;83(6):1178–82. https://doi.org/10.4269/ajtmh.2010.10-0527.
5. Jogerst K, Callender B, Adams V, et al. Identifying interprofessional global health competencies for 21st-century health professionals. Ann Glob Health. 2015;81(2):239–47. https://doi.org/10.1016/j.aogh.2015.03.006.
6. Pancheshnikov A, Cuneo CN, Matias WR, et al. Case studies in adaptation: centring equity in global health education during the COVID-19 pandemic and beyond. BMJ Glob Health. 2023;8(4):e011682. https://doi.org/10.1136/bmjgh-2023-011682.

Chapter 47
5-Year and 10-Year Plans

Alexander Santangelo and Robin Perry

All transitions in life can be both stressful and exciting; the transition from resident to attending is no different. The paths available to us are endless, which is wonderful and perhaps a bit frightening. This book has numerous sections to provide ideas and guidance for a number of different paths that an obstetrician gynecologist could aspire to walk down. But how do we realistically manage to achieve these aspirations with all the competing interests in our lives? This chapter provides helpful suggestions on how to maintain direction and focus through the process of forming your own 5-year and 10-year plan.

Why Have a Plan?

Creating and maintaining a 5- or 10-year plan, or life plan, can be a beneficial exercise. It leads to a better understanding of ourselves, where we are at the moment, and what changes could be made to lead to a more fulfilling and well-rounded life [1]. The resulting product of completing a life plan includes a list of goals, plans to achieve them, and a rough timetable. Completing a life plan can help you identify gaps and provide motivation and the confidence to start taking action toward a future that is more fulfilling to us and those we hold dear.

A. Santangelo (✉)
Division of Research, Department of Obstetrics and Gynecology, Cooper University Health Care, Camden, NJ, USA

R. Perry
Division of Maternal-Fetal Medicine, Department of Obstetrics and Gynecology, Cooper Medical School of Rowan University and Cooper University Health Care, Camden, NJ, USA

A. Malik et al. (eds.), *An Obstetrician/Gynecologist's Path*,
https://doi.org/10.1007/978-3-031-87098-9_47

How to Start: Introspection and Feedback

Life plans are deeply personal and unique to every individual. For that reason, a great first step toward creating a life plan is to actively work on better understanding ourselves. Self-awareness is the ability to see yourself clearly and objectively, which is not easily accomplished. It can be achieved through introspection and reflection. Spending the time to work toward self-awareness will help ensure that the life plan we develop leads us somewhere that is meaningful and fulfilling. Although it might seem basic, it is very worthwhile, particularly for those who are very busy, to spend time reflecting on who we are.

A meaningful life plan should have goals that reflect what is important to us. Motley and McMullin [2] describe a helpful 5-point framework for identifying what is important in life: (1) Mission & Identity, (2) Direction, (3) Family, (4) Fun, and (5) Finances. This is a useful way to conceptualize and guide our reflection on who we are and eventually the creation of our goals. Below are some questions that can help us explore what is important to consider when making a life plan based on these five categories.

- Mission and Identity
  - What helps me maintain my core identity?
  - What makes me feel fulfilled or accomplished?
  - What values are important for me to maintain?
  - What are the issues in life that I am most passionate about?
- Direction
  - What does a more fulfilled version of myself look like?
  - What are my areas of weakness that I want to avoid?
  - Where are my strengths that I can capitalize on?
  - Where do I want my career to go?
    - Do I want to pursue a fellowship or another degree?
    - Do I want to work in a private practice after working in an academic practice?
  - What does success look like to me?
- Family
  - Who are the people I want close to me in my life, and how do I want that to look?
  - Do I want to be partnered or married?
  - Do I want children, and what do I need to support that family?
- Fun
  - What brings me joy or makes me smile?
  - What interests or activities make time seem to fly by?

  - What does a perfect day of work look like to me?
- Finances
  - For the life I want to lead, what will I need to budget for?
  - How much work do I need to do to cover my expenses/budget?
  - Over what period of time do I want to pay off my student loans?
  - When will I retire and what do I need to do now to prepare?

As an exercise, try free writing or dictating about these topics. Use what you create to guide your reflections. You do not have to answer every question, nor do you have to write anything down. Some prefer to take time for quiet contemplation and work through the concepts in their minds. You also might find it helpful to consider this exercise during your regular self-care routine, while exercising, meditating, practicing yoga, etc.

Next, utilize those close to you as sounding boards to get external perspectives on yourself. Soliciting true and honest feedback from trusted friends, family, and colleagues can be an eye-opening process. Select these people carefully and be purposeful when choosing what questions to ask each person. Remember that the goal of asking these questions is to gain insight into yourself, not to identify barriers or other people's goals for you. Use the thoughts on and answers to these questions to help inform you on the next step in the process, identifying your mission, vision, and goals.

Personal Mission Statement

Our personal mission statement describes our purpose, core values, and principles that guide us throughout life. For many, our personal mission is influenced by the reasons we worked so hard to become an obstetrician gynecologist. Our mission is also tied very closely to our personal identity and the values that guide us to the actions that we take day to day. A personal mission statement could look like this:

> To provide equitable, culturally competent care to a diverse and underserved population, while working to empower this population to advocate for their care needs.

Personal Vision Statement

Considering our thoughts about what is important to us and the direction we desire for our career path, we can develop our own personal vision statement. The vision statement should provide a big-picture perspective and clarify long-term aspirations. Our personal vision statement should feel inspiring and motivational. A personal vision statement could look like this:

I will become a respected regional leader in quality healthcare for women, developing a large group practice that prioritizes advocacy for women, quality care and patient satisfaction.

Goals and Objectives

After spending the time needed to consider the more abstract concepts used to develop our mission and vision statements, it is time to specify the more concrete goals and objectives needed to develop our life plan. Goals are broad outcomes that we want to achieve or general intentions that we have. When identifying and writing out our goals, we should always keep our personal vision statement in mind and ensure that these goals will help us to walk down a path toward that vision. Many of us will have concrete goals that we know we want to accomplish in the future, like passing our written and oral board exams to become board certified in our specialty and subspecialty. However, not all goals are that concrete. For example, we may want to explore or work to gain knowledge and experience in an area like pediatric gynecology or alternative medicine. These would absolutely be appropriate goals.

Once we have our goals identified, we know what it is that we want to accomplish. The next step is to list our objectives for each of our goals. Our objectives are the defined actions that we need to accomplish to achieve our larger goal. When developing objectives, it can be helpful to use SMART objectives, which ask us to ensure that each objective is specific, measurable, achievable, relevant, and time-bound [3]. Below are a few example goals and SMART objectives a new obstetrician gynecologist attending may have.

5-Year Goal Examples

To clarify the process of developing SMART objectives, each SMART element has been listed for the first example goal.

Example 1
Goal: "To hone my clinical skills and expertise as a new attending Obstetrician Gynecologist."

Objective 1: Complete at least 20 minimally invasive hysterectomies within my first 2 years as an attending.

- Specific The objective identifies the exact types of surgeries to track.
- Measurable Tracked as total surgeries through quarterly EMR or billing reports.
- Achievable The objective is possible based on the caseload of my practice.

- Relevant — Completing these surgeries will increase my gynecologic surgical skills.
- Time-bound — I have 2 years to accomplish this.

Objective 2: I will treat at least 100 new obstetric patients in my clinic in my first year of practice.

- Specific — The objective states what type of experience is needed.
- Measurable — Total number of visits can be tracked using EMR reports.
- Achievable — The visit total is within the average of my practice and schedule.
- Relevant — Treating new obstetric patients will help me to perfect my ambulatory office skills.
- Time-bound — I have a deadline of 1 year from my start date.

Example 2
Goal: "To build professional relationships and begin networking in the Obstetrics and Gynecology community."

Objective 1: Identify and attend four regional conferences over the next 3 years.
Objective 2: Pre-register for the next upcoming national conference in my specialty by the end of the month.
Objective 3: Join two professional organizations that nurture my sense of mission in the next 3 months.
Objective 4: Initiate a collaborative project with a colleague within the next year so I can have a poster to submit at a national conference 2 years from now.

10-Year Goal Examples

From a 10-year perspective, things look different. Goals like passing our boards and gaining clinical expertise fall way to goals with a broader scope like owning property, having a positive reputation in the community you serve, and building your CV.

Example 1
Goal: "Move into a house in an area with good elementary schools for my children which is within commuting distance for my partner and I."

Objective 1: Over the next year, identify areas/neighborhoods of interest and townships that meet the location requirements of my family and me.
Objective 2: Create a family budget within the next 6 months that allows adequate savings for a down payment.
Objective 3: Decide on what aspects of a home are most important to my partner and me and have a shared running list until we meet a realtor.
Objective 4: Improve my overall credit rating over the next 2 years by hiring a trusted credit repair group.

Example 2
Goal: "Begin my journey on the academic track and become an Associate Professor."

Objective 1: Have five first-authored, peer-reviewed academic products within the next 4 years when I am eligible for academic promotion.
Objective 2: Volunteer as a reviewer for the Green Journal this year and review at least two articles per year.
Objective 3: Demonstrate my leadership skills by serving as Chair of at least one hospital committee and one medical school committee over the next 4 years.
Objective 4: Serve on at least one national committee over the next 2 years.
Objective 5: Apply for at least ten federally funded research grant over the next 8 years.

When thinking about more long-term goals, some people may find a benefit from going further and defining even smaller steps as sub-objectives under the more daunting objectives of the plan. The sub-objectives can be used to create a checklist. Other people find that this level of detail distracts from the larger vision that they want to keep in mind. Find a level of detail that provides structure and works for you while not being overwhelming.

Be Flexible

Keep in mind that life plans are not concrete. Interests, priorities, family dynamics, and societal trends can all change, causing your personal vision to evolve. It is important to know that non-adherence to a plan is not a failure, it is a part of personal growth, which is natural. Creating a life plan is an exercise that helps to define long-term goals and identify the smaller objectives that can be accomplished to help achieve them. This is a process that can motivate and empower. The benefits of creating and having a life plan do not come from strictly and perfectly following the plan, but instead they come from the process of introspection and identification of concrete steps that can provide focus and direction.

References

1. McNevin M. How to develop a 5-year career plan. Harvard Business Review. 27 Sept 2023. https://hbr.org/2023/09/how-to-develop-a-5-year-career-plan. Accessed on 5 Feb 2024.
2. Motley RJ, McMullin A. Developing your professional career plan. Fam Pract Manag. 2020;27(4):21–4.
3. Doran GT. There's a SMART way to write management's goals and objectives. J Manag Rev. 1981;70:35–6.

Part V
Maintaining Your Health

Chapter 48
Starting a Family

Amanda Malik

"There's never a good time to have a baby" is such a classic line that I'm sure everyone reading this chapter has heard it. In many ways, it's true—a career in medicine is demanding and time intensive, and certainly a naysayer can come up with a list of disadvantages to childbearing at any point in your career. To many, this statement may seem daunting—if there's never a good time, when to consider it? However, I'd argue that it can be freeing. There may not ever be a "good" time; therefore, you don't have to delay indefinitely. The best time to have a baby is when *you* are ready. While starting a family is ultimately such a personal decision that I could not possibly cover all situations, hypothetical or otherwise, in this chapter, I do attempt to offer one Ob/Gyn's perspective and introspection about the family planning process. While I am not so confident to believe that I have the answers, there are a few interactions through the years regarding family planning that stuck with me, and so this chapter relies on the experiences of others (from my perspective) as well.

Very early in medical school, one of my classmates got pregnant. She was understandably nervous and kept it under wraps for a little while until we were doing an immersive week in the hospital. She wasn't having the easiest pregnancy, and so observing long ICU rounds and surgeries, even without being scrubbed in, was tough. When she revealed to a group of us that she was expecting, I remember worrying for her about the timing. A baby, at the beginning of medical school! I had barely enough time to take care of myself, let alone another being (and one who keeps you up many hours of the night). Remarkably, she delivered during one of the last blocks of the year, took a short period off, and then used the summer to catch up on the block she had missed. She was an incredible mom right away; her own mother helped her care for the baby and often brought her to the school so she could

A. Malik (✉)
Department of Obstetrics and Gynecology, Cooper Medical School of Rowan University and Cooper University Health Care, Camden, NJ, USA

A. Malik et al. (eds.), *An Obstetrician/Gynecologist's Path*,
https://doi.org/10.1007/978-3-031-87098-9_48

breastfeed in between lectures. Her newborn daughter quickly became a beloved addition and mascot of sorts for our class. While I couldn't have imagined having a baby at the onset of medical school, I later found myself fantasizing about having a newborn without the restrictions of clinical responsibilities that come later in medical school and residency.

As a second-year medical student, I attended a panel of women physicians about being a female in medicine. The planned questions focused on various forms of discrimination, work life balance, and advancing opportunities, without directly addressing fertility. However, a brave plastic surgery fellow who was on the panel took a question about family planning and opened up to the audience about her fertility struggles. She had started medical school a few years after college, went on to residency and fellowship, and thought about having a baby as her fellowship wrapped up. I don't remember the exact circumstances, but after trying to conceive naturally, she sought assistance from REI and was told she could not conceive. It sounds to my Ob/Gyn brain now like premature ovarian insufficiency, but at the time the specific diagnosis did not matter; what stood out was the deep pain she felt and the urgency with which she advised the female audience about the risks of waiting too long.

Personally, I began to feel ready to start a family in my second year of residency. I got married in October and was initially looking forward to more international trips with my husband after getting through the slog of intern year. Then COVID-19 hit and halted all my daydreaming. Perhaps it was spending all the time at home that shifted my mindset, or perhaps it was some biological clock, as I also turned 30 that year. Whatever it was, I started thinking about starting a family seriously. After some angst and soliciting advice from a former chief resident who had a baby during my intern year, my husband and I decided to start trying. It took nearly a year—with a brief pause during the months that would have set my due date for June or July—but I got pregnant, worked until 39 weeks, and with the blessing of the ARRIVE trial, scheduled an elective induction at 39w0d, during August of my chief year.

Having a baby during residency is not for the faint of heart. I was grateful to have 6 weeks off, though I simultaneously realized how inadequate that time was. I was lucky to have a partner who got more time off, as well as family who stepped up to help with childcare even on some very early mornings and very late nights. On those long days I missed my baby, and more than once shed some tears standing over him sleeping in his crib as I realized I had missed all his awake hours that day. I did my best to make up for that whenever I could, by being fully present when I was home, using vacation time to just be a mom, and taking some extra time off between finishing residency and starting my attending job. I never regretted my decision to have a baby in residency, as I was ready to be a mom and felt so fulfilled by taking on that new role.

I had my second baby just short of 1 year after starting my attending job. I hadn't yet taken the ABOG certifying exam or really fully established myself in my career, but again, I was ready. In many ways having a baby after residency was easier—in my state with generous parental leave I got much more time off, and was actually sleeping several consecutive hours by the time I went back to work. Still, it had its own challenges—I worried about being able to pick up my surgical skills again and feared I wouldn't have a panel of patients who continued to see me annually if they had to wait several additional months for me or had to see one of my partners in the interim. Both of these things worked out. I made sure not to delay any pending surgeries after I returned from leave and picked up cases from non-operating partners; I was also pleasantly surprised to see patients who had delayed their annual a few months to continue their care with me. Again, I didn't regret my timing, as I had been ready to expand my family.

I was lucky to have relatively easy pregnancies, but I'd be remiss if I didn't acknowledge the possible difficulties that can occur. Even as the field of medicine surpasses the 50/50 barrier, with more women enrolling in medical school than men [1], and even as participants in a field that's becoming dominated by women [2], there can be barriers to starting a family. Medical training is notoriously long and arduous, facts I don't have to emphasize to anyone reading this book. Recent studies have highlighted that female surgeons have significantly higher rates of miscarriage than the general population; are more likely to delay having children and more likely to use assisted reproductive technology (ART); and are more likely to have major pregnancy complications, especially when operating 12 or more hours a week during the third trimester [3] (a number easily met by many still in training). These challenges are exacerbated by a lack of formal fertility education in many specialties, limited parental leave policies (with limited transparency), and typically no support financially or hourly for elective oocyte preservation [4]. The fact that studies highlighting these challenges exist is encouraging; for most of modern medical training, no one was even researching this. New programs offering financial support for residents desiring oocyte preservation, models to prevent overnight call in the third trimester, and ACGME requirements for parental leave are promising, but realistically, widely available solutions are still a ways off.

You may have started reading this chapter because you, too, are feeling ready to have a baby or grow your family. If you are, I encourage you to follow that feeling and pursue your personal goals as well as your career goals. While some advanced planning and shoring up support can certainly make the process easier, remember there may not be any good time to have a baby—so the best time is when you are ready.

References

1. Boyle P. More women than men are enrolled in medical school. AAMC News. 2019. https://www.aamc.org/news/more-women-men-are-enrolled-medical-school.
2. Vassar L. How medical specialties vary by gender. AMA Specialty Profiles. 2015. https://www.ama-assn.org/medical-students/specialty-profiles/how-medical-specialties-vary-gender.
3. Rangel EL, Castillo-Angeles M, Easter SR, et al. Incidence of infertility and pregnancy complications in US female surgeons. JAMA Surg. 2021;156(10):905–15. https://doi.org/10.1001/jamasurg.2021.3301.
4. Hayden H, et al. Decreased fertility awareness amongst surgeons and surgical trainees and potential role of formal fertility education. J Surg Educ. 2024;81(7):947–59. https://doi.org/10.1016/j.jsurg.2024.03.011.

Chapter 49
Maintaining Personal Health and Family Life

Michelle Iavicoli

Introduction

"Work life balance." A buzz word in popular culture. As a resident, did you embrace this? Many students and young health care professionals are seduced by the tireless hours of medical intrigue that the medical field has to offer, ignoring a sense of balance. But the importance of work-life balance cannot be discounted. Finding a work life balance after residency is essential to maintain a healthy sustainable career that balances work, personal health, and family. Finding this balance will make for better quality of patient care and a more rewarding sustainable career. Let's explore some crucial elements of health essential to fostering your own health and your relationship with your family.

Personal Health

Physical Health

Start with the basics. Practice what you preach! Establish healthy habits from the beginning with your exercise, sleep, and diet. The CDC recommends 150 minutes a week of aerobic exercise and at least two sessions of muscle strengthening exercises per week [1]. Start to incorporate this routine from day one. Schedule your personal health time on your calendar so that it is protected time. Once this becomes part of

M. Iavicoli (✉)
Department of Obstetrics and Gynecology, Cooper Medical School of Rowan University and Cooper University Health Care, Camden, NJ, USA

A. Malik et al. (eds.), *An Obstetrician/Gynecologist's Path*,
https://doi.org/10.1007/978-3-031-87098-9_49

your routine, no one will take away your "me time." Make time to sleep. It is recommended that adults sleep 7–9 hours per night [2]. Studies show that getting less than that may promote several health issues including cardiovascular, hormonal, metabolic, and cognitive issues [3]. Make every effort to maximize your time at work; equally important is to know when to shut it down and rest. Not only will you be a better provider, but a more efficient and effective provider.

You are what you eat! Take time to have meals. Abandon the practice of eating on the run, in the car, while walking around the hospital. Chances are your diet will be higher in calories, higher fat, and higher in carbs than a meal that you take the time to prepare, sit down and eat. If time is a constraint, plan your meals on the weekend. Precook when you have time off. Bring all your meals and snacks to work so the time you eat will be yours. Bring your own healthy snacks to avoid the unhealthy snacks often found in the work room or common area. In the end, you will feel better about yourself avoiding the sugar highs and lows.

Mental Health

Just like the patients we treat, we can experience depression, anxiety, and fatigue. It is equally important for us to maintain a balance of our emotional well-being to best care for your patients. It begins with awareness. Physicians can be prone to mental health issues given the high level of stress, the long clinical hours, financial burdens, and inability to balance work and home life. Clinicians often do not seek help for a variety of reasons. Ego, stigma, and concerns for confidentiality often prevent physicians from seeking help when needed. Start simple. Start to develop coping techniques now. Adopt mindfulness; engage friends, family, and colleagues support; and practice relaxation techniques now. Awareness and prevention are key to maintaining a healthy balance of your mental health.

Family Life

You have your work family, but your personal family deserves equal time. Make time for them. Your family may be your pet, siblings, parents, partners, or children. Each plays a significant role in your life. They will support you, but they need your time in return. Carving out family time from your busy schedule will allow you to be more physically and mentally strong. Share your schedule with your family so they have realistic expectations around your availability. Schedule dedicated time to spend with them. It is truly quality time they will value and remember not quantity. Always strive to provide them with your undivided attention. Put away your cell phone. Turn off the computer. Quality time is not time spent watching TV together while you close your charts. I recently asked my adult children if they felt slighted as I worked during their upbringing while many of their friends had stay-at-home parents. My daughter quickly responded "no mom because when you were home you spent your time with us, doing fun things. That is my memory." It is reassurance that quality time wins over quantity.

Consumed with the rigors of a new career, new hospital, and new partners, when is the best time to start your family? There is no right answer. Simply start it when it feels right for you and your partner. Don't start your family simply because of your age or because you feel pressure that all your friends already have children. Medicine is a unique career path that often can delay family planning. Make sure you feel settled with your new position before you add another layer of stress by starting or growing your family. In contrast, don't feel bad about expanding your family right away! Your colleagues expect you will start your family or grow your family if you haven't done so yet. Don't feel guilty. They will cover for you, just as you will cover for them. Proceed when it is the right time for you. Is there life after children?

Planning for the Future

Maintaining your personal health not only requires daily maintenance, but it necessitates planning for your future well-being too. Find a balance between your work life and your family life. Will the physical and mental demands of your career be sustainable or do you need to think about branching your career interests. Get involved with administration, engage in quality work, take on a role with education either of students or residents. Not only will this add a layer of fulfillment to your career now, but it will also afford you an area to rebalance your career in the future. Plan for life after kids. Your children won't need you forever. Establish your own hobbies and interests so when your kids are grown, you and your partner have interests other than those revolving around your children. Take up a hobby, learn to play golf, start a garden, take up painting. Hobbies and interests out of work will allow a balance in your life while working and will extend through retirement. Time and again, I witness aging providers afraid to retire because they don't know what they will do with their free time. Plan now and engage in activities outside of medicine. This will allow you a more balanced career, and a smooth transition into retirement.

Conclusion

Maintaining your personal health and family life beyond residency takes work and dedication. Take care of your personal health, both physical and mental. Dedicate quality time to your family and loved ones. Share your schedule with your partner and family. Engage in shared responsibility. Plan for your future well-being too. Your personal well-being will directly affect you, your family, friends, patients, and colleagues. Engage it and maintain it to the best of your ability. Doing this will carry you through a very meaningful, balanced career.

References

1. American Heart Association. How much physical activity do you need? www.heart.org. https://www.heart.org/en/healthy-living/fitness/fitness-basics/aha-recs-for-physical-activity-infographic. 16 Mar 2021.
2. U.S. Department of Health and Human Services. Why is sleep important? National Heart Lung and Blood Institute. https://www.nhlbi.nih.gov/health/sleep/why-sleep-important. 22 Mar 2022.
3. U.S. Department of Health and Human Services. How much sleep is enough? National Heart Lung and Blood Institute. https://www.nhlbi.nih.gov/health/sleep/how-much-sleep. 22 Mar 2022.

Chapter 50
Preventing Burnout

Michelle Iavicoli

Introduction

When you enter medicine, you are eager, excited, and full of enthusiasm! Long days and nights of medical studies start to wear you down. Long days in the hospital sap your enthusiasm and begin to make you callous and jaded. What happened in that short period of time? You are beginning to feel the early signs of burnout. But you still have your entire career ahead of you! How can signs of burnout creep into your daily life so prematurely? Well, burnout is real. Without understanding burnout, it is difficult to prevent or manage. In this chapter, let's explore what burnout really is, how to prevent it, and how to manage it and reverse it. Establishing tools to prevent burnout early in your career will allow for a more meaningful, satisfying career. It begins with understanding, what is burnout?

What Is Burnout?

Burnout is defined as "physical, emotional or mental exhaustion accompanied by a decreased motivation, lowering performance and a negative attitude toward oneself and others" [1]. It is not uncommon that one's self-awareness of signs of burnout is ignored or unrecognized. High workload and long hours set a foundation for burnout in medicine. Are you short with your patients, cranky to your significant other, snippy towards your staff? These may be early signs of burnout. A provider's workload may not consist of only patient care. It may be layered with administrative

M. Iavicoli (✉)
Department of Obstetrics and Gynecology, Cooper Medical School of Rowan University and Cooper University Health Care, Camden, NJ, USA

A. Malik et al. (eds.), *An Obstetrician/Gynecologist's Path*,
https://doi.org/10.1007/978-3-031-87098-9_50

duties, scheduling, quality and safety work, educational responsibilities, in addition to personal life obligations. This compiled stress can lead to anger, detachment, and even complacency in your responsibilities. The nature of our work often places us in high stress, quick decision circumstances that can also mount stress and be emotionally draining. A ruptured ectopic pregnancy, a severe postpartum hemorrhage, a category three fetal tracing, all these clinical scenarios add mounted stress to our workload, contributing to burnout. Recognizing these signs early on will hopefully help to prevent or reverse your progression to burnout. What tools do we have to prevent getting to this stage of burnout in medicine?

How to Prevent Burnout?

The prevention of burnout begins with self-assessment. Do I manage my time well? Am I capable of accepting additional work responsibilities like additional resident coverage, student lectures, chairing a safety committee, or staffing a community event? If you feel constantly overwhelmed, keep a calendar and don't overlap your obligations. Book your personal time first then layer on your work and extracurricular activities related to work. Learn to say no when it is simply not practical to take on an additional task. In the long run, you will be respected for being realistic and honest, rather than completing something late and incomplete or poorly completed. This is where prevention of burnout begins.

Always make time for yourself. Self-care is crucial in preventing burnout. Make time to sleep, eat, and exercise. Schedule time with your family and friends. A social life is as valuable to your mental health as exercise is to your physical health. It is this balance that will bring you happiness and balance and prevent burnout.

If you feel yourself spiraling towards burnout, take a critical look at what is bringing you down. Learn some coping strategies for dealing with stress. Coping strategies could include deep breathing, mindfulness, or exercise. Seek a strong mentor to guide you and challenge you to develop means to cope with high stress situations. Ask for feedback, am I coping and balancing well or is there room for improvement? Sometimes an objective eye will see much more clearly mistakes that you are making that may lead to burnout.

Rely on your family, friends, and colleagues to build a supportive network. At times only your colleagues will understand the nature of the day-to-day stresses that an obstetrician experiences. It may be a partner who encourages you to take time to exercise or eat well when you are overloaded with work. A best friend may be the only one that senses you are spiraling into an emotionally fragile state. Your supportive network collectively will be your rock at times when you are most vulnerable. Lean on them equally and engage them as vital components of your well-being, helping you to prevent burnout during your career.

Will There be an Occasion When You Admit Burnout?

Likely so but learning to deal with burnout will make you a more resilient physician who ultimately sees a more sustainable career in medicine. Dealing with burnout will require a multifaceted approach. Start with engaging your support network. Are your colleagues also experiencing similar feelings of burnout? Could the workload be distributed or shared? Are you engaging in menial tasks and not prioritizing those that are most important? How are they handling the stresses of the job? Often your peers have valuable insight into workload, balance, and sustainability. Learn from them. By sharing with them, your collaboration will help not only you but them as well.

Ask for professional help. Whether it be mental health support, stress management programs, or professional counseling. You may need more tools to help you cope when times are difficult. Seek out trained professionals. No one will ever fault you for admitting you are down, but they will fault you for acknowledging you have signs of burnout yet refusing to seek support.

Lean on your family. They know you well. Listen to their cues. Is your partner asking why you are always negative and grumpy towards the family? Maybe they know you best and perceive signs of burnout in you. They may play an integral part in your recovery. Spend time with them. Engage in self-care with them. Use them as sounding boards. Your family may provide the greatest strength in reversing your burnout because they know you best. They know what brings you down and what ultimately will bring you back to balance within your career and home life. Use them wisely.

This multidisciplinary approach, utilizing colleagues, professionals, and family members will redirect you in times of burnout back on a more balanced track in your professional career.

Conclusion

Burnout is real! As a new obstetrician you are starting out ahead of your peers if you understand what burnout is, how to prevent it, and when it hits how to deal with it. Be proactive to develop tools to prevent burnout in your career. Find that balance in your work-life and develop coping strategies to deal stress when it hits. Always prioritize self-care and lean on those around you. When burnout hits, rebalance yourself with the tools you are given to get back on track. Following this model will hopefully allow you to enjoy a productive, balanced sustainable career in obstetrics.

Reference

1. American Psychological Association. APA dictionary of psychology. American Psychological Association. https://dictionary.apa.org/burnout. 19 Apr 2018.

Chapter 51
Divorce

Michelle Iavicoli

Introduction

No one ever thinks they will have to endure something as traumatic as divorce. Unfortunately, even the best marriages sometimes end up in divorce. When you need to navigate divorce, you should be prepared personally, professionally, financially, and legally to handle it. Yes, there is life after divorce, although going through it may seem incomprehensible.

Personally

As obstetricians, we are expected to provide emotional stability for our patients, often counseling them on delicate subjects such as pregnancy loss, infertility, and infidelity. When facing a divorce, we are faced with the same emotional upheaval often experienced by our patients. It may be the most impactful event in a provider's career. This emotional upheaval often manifests as stress. Stress can be felt in the workplace, at home with family and with friends. Don't forget to use your tools for stress reduction. Take time to take care of yourself both mentally and physically. Practice mindfulness, exercise, eat, and sleep as best as you can. Total body health will maintain both your physical and mental strength while getting through this difficult time. Emotionally you may navigate the stages of grief, denial, anger, bargaining, depression, and acceptance. Rely on your support system to navigate each

M. Iavicoli (✉)
Department of Obstetrics and Gynecology, Cooper Medical School of Rowan University and Cooper University Health Care, Camden, NJ, USA

A. Malik et al. (eds.), *An Obstetrician/Gynecologist's Path*,
https://doi.org/10.1007/978-3-031-87098-9_51

stage. Be careful not to take these emotions into the workplace as it may impact the quality of care that you provide for your patients.

Professionally

Divorce may impact your professional life as an obstetrician. You may need to alter your schedule to meet with attorneys or to meet the demands of altered childcare. You may have less flexibility in your daily schedule and be unable to stay late to add on that extra patient or finish the delivery you have started. This can ultimately affect the quality of your care that you provide. Do the best that you can to provide quality over quantity of care. Reassure yourself that this is temporary, and you will adjust for your new demands in your schedule. Lean on your colleagues, they too will face challenges during their career and you in turn will support them.

Maintain your privacy and dignity. Your colleagues, patients, and staff will be aware that you are navigating a challenging time in your life. Engage them for support but keep the details private. Your dignity lies on the laurels of your grace and poise in this time of crisis. Hold your head high, be strong, and in moments of weakness engage their help, they will be there for you.

Financially

Don't let divorce destroy you financially. You have invested numerous years and dollars into this career in medicine. Don't blow it all away on a divorce. Do engage a competent attorney who has your best interest in mind. Do support your absolute needs but be flexible. The more you dispute, the more money you both will lose to the attorneys. When possible, use a mediator, agree upon what you can mutually and pay attorney fees for what remain absolute sticking points. There is no reason why the attorney should end up with most of your assets. Alimony and child support can add an additional level of stress to your financial contract. Often professionals find themselves moonlighting to supplement new financial obligations. Be mindful to not allow divorce to compromise your financial stability.

Life After Divorce

Many professionals find it hard to see their future post-divorce. As an emotionally and physically draining experience with financial complexity, life after divorce seems impossible. Good news is life goes on. Agreements will be made, possessions will be split, children will adjust, and life will go on. So will your profession. In fact, don't forget to embrace your career while going through these difficult times of divorce. It is the stability of your work; getting up every morning, dressing, speaking to colleagues and patients that is the best routine around. Stability and consistency will help you to heal. Keep going to work, engage your colleagues, make small talk with your patients. This will be the best therapy that you could buy! When it is over, move on. Don't lament the past. Make new routines and hobbies. Engage new friends or interests inside and out of work. Change may not only be good for you but make you a more rounded individual. Keep believing in and growing you.

Conclusion

Divorce is complex and challenging to navigate. No one signs up for marriage thinking someday they will divorce. It can be an unfortunate reality of life. Being prepared for the personal, professional, and financial impact that divorce brings will give you the tools needed to navigate divorce in a dignified and respectful manner.

Chapter 52
Mindfulness

Karissa Rajagopal

> A lot of times I've had to pretend I felt good when I felt terrible.
> —Venus Williams

While we cannot control so much of what happens in our day-to-day practice, we can control how we respond to it. Practicing mindfulness can help us stay sane in the face of chaotic life as an OBGYN. I have no formal training or credentials in this topic. Prior to residency, I considered myself a happy and healthy person. I laughed a lot, exercised daily, and ate a well-balanced diet. During my intern year, despite biking 3 miles to and from work and eating the most vegetables out of all the residents combined, I still developed hypertension and depression. Terrified of the trajectory of my health and career path, I began to try to understand what is it about our specialty that makes us one of the leaders in burnout, depression, and suicide and how I can prevent that for myself. Through this chapter, I will share my current findings and practices.

Our duty to our patients and desire to improve their well-being consistently supersedes our own. We often ignore our own basic bodily needs. We miss major moments in our friends' and family's lives. We develop strong attachments to our patients and experience terrible losses. We then take all of these emotions and shove them down as far as possible so we can move on to the next task [1].

K. Rajagopal (✉)
Department of Obstetrics and Gynecology, Cooper Medical School of Rowan University and Cooper University Health Care, Camden, NJ, USA

A. Malik et al. (eds.), *An Obstetrician/Gynecologist's Path*,
https://doi.org/10.1007/978-3-031-87098-9_52

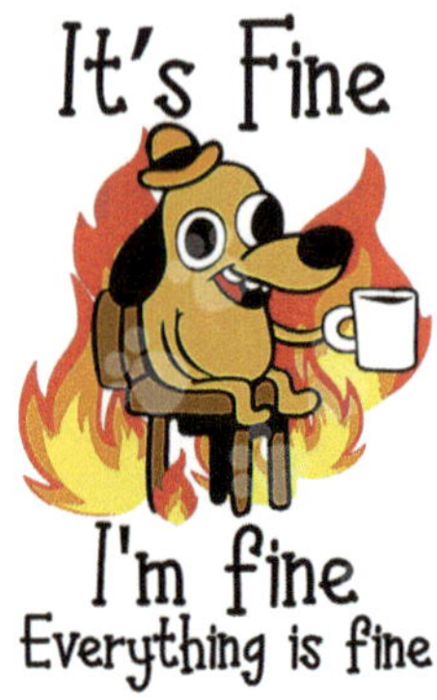

Source: The meme
'This is fine' creator reflects on 10 years of the comic meme: NPR
https://www.npr.org/2023/01/16/1149232763/this-is-fine-meme-anniversary-gunshow-web-comic

In this chapter, through the practice of mindfulness, we will discuss ways to clear the mind so that we can have room to identify our emotions. "It is through identification and acknowledgment of one's feelings that we will begin to gain insight to ameliorate our own forms of suffering. Otherwise, if we continue to go through life being stressed while not knowing we are stressed, there is little we can do to protect ourselves from the long-term physiological consequences." —Garbor Matte

Mindfulness has no single definition, but the definition that has helped me is the receptive attention and awareness of current events and experiences [2]. This entails acknowledging our own thoughts and emotions as they arise—while also accepting external stimuli without assigning inherent meaning. This frame of thinking is often referred to as "decentering." It encourages a broader awareness, to view thoughts as thoughts, and observations as observations. This allows space for mental distance/disengagement from situations and increases the capacity to be present for others' thoughts, emotions, and needs. It can decrease biased personal memories, learned associations, or future projections.

The two most studied meditation-based clinical programs are modeled on well-known stress reduction practices: the relaxation response (RR) program developed by Herbert Benson and the mindfulness-based stress reduction (MBSR) program developed by Jon Kabat-Zinn [3]. The RR program is designed to counteract the stress response by targeting relaxation and reducing arousal and muscle tension across the body, aiming to decrease sympathetic activation. In contrast, the primary goal of the MBSR program is to cultivate mindfulness by directing attention to present-moment and sensory experiences throughout the body, without attempting to alter anything [4].

Given physicians' demanding schedules, their availability to attend mindfulness programs or yoga classes is often limited. The main objective of this chapter is to offer an introduction to mindfulness and suggestions on how to incorporate mindfulness into a busy schedule. Of course, mindfulness is not a one size fits all. Practices and effectiveness will vary among individuals. There is no single correct way to be mindful. The first section will explore methods to "check in" with the mind, body, and environment, whereas part 2 will focus on incorporating bodywork and meditation practices into a busy schedule.

Part 1: Checking In

Checking in with the Mind: Am I in Fight or Flight vs Rest and Digest?

Physicians frequently navigate high-stress environments. Even during the moments of apparent tranquility, looming responsibilities still linger in the background. Due to the multitude of challenges, physicians often find themselves in a perpetual state of "fight or flight" mode. This involves a continuous heightened physiological and psychological arousal linked to the body's stress response. The sympathetic nervous system takes the lead-releasing stress hormonesraising blood pressure and heart rate and tensing muscles. The insidious and constant chronic stress affects both mental and physical health [5]. It is during the fight or flight mode that individuals may be more prone to snapping at coworkers, experiencing heightened frustration due to delays in cases, or feeling overwhelmed by workload. Alternatively, rest and digest refers to activating the parasympathetic nervous system, which promotes relaxation, digestion, and other essential bodily functions when the body is at rest [5].

Returning to the definition of mindfulness, receptive attention, and awareness of current events and experiences, understanding which subconscious autonomic processes are occurring can provide insight into the present state of the mind.

Reflective Questions

- Am I experiencing a fight response (body tightening, verbal impulse, raised voice, feeling anger, urge to confront, urge to do the opposite of what others are doing)?
- Am I experiencing a flight response (restlessness, lack of focus, feeling trapped, trouble responding, anxiety in body, shifting attention)?
- What is the underlying cause of this response today?

Checking in with the Body: Once I Am Still, What Hurts?

After a long day standing in an OR, running around the clinic, OBGYNs know too well the sensation of an aching sensation in every muscle and the throbbing sensation in their feet and calves. A body scan is a common mindful practice that involves systematically directing attention to different parts of the body, typically from head to toe or vice versa. During a body scan, individuals are guided to bring their attention to each part of the body, noticing sensations, tension, or discomfort without judgment or the need to change anything [6].

The process of a body scan typically involves the following steps:

1. Settle into a comfortable position: Lie flat in a relaxed position (can also be done sitting or standing).
2. Bring attention to the breath: Take a few seconds or minutes of focusing on the breath to settle the mind and body.
3. Systematically scan the body: Start from the top of the head or the tips of the toes, attention is directed to each part of the body sequentially IE scalp, forehead, eyesbrows, jaw, neck, shoulders, arms, hands, fingers, knuckles, chest, ribs abdomen, hips, legs, feet, and toes.
4. Notice sensations: Notice any sensations present, such as warmth, coolness, tingling, tension, or relaxation. Observe sensations as they are, without trying to change them or attach labels to them.
5. Release tension: If tension or discomfort is noticed in any area, bring gentle awareness and acceptance to that sensation, allowing it to soften or release naturally.
6. Cultivate awareness: The goal is to maintain present-moment awareness of the body and sensations, gently returning attention to the body whenever the mind wanders.

Reflection Questions

- What joints hurt today?
- What muscles did I use most today?
- What position did I spend most of my day in?

Checking in with the Environment: Do My Surroundings Nourish or Drain Me?

Workspaces often accumulate a variety of items, from old patient charts to lingering birthday decorations to unread medical journals. Amid the demands of patient care, it becomes convenient to clear a small area by the computer and dive into work.

However, the presence of these extra objects can impact stress levels and the cognitive load associated with overstimulation.

Intentional space management involves consciously organizing and designing your environment to support well-being, enhance productivity, and foster mindfulness. This concept is intricately connected to the notion that your physical surroundings can significantly influence your mental health. Exploring intentional space practices can yield several benefits for mental health and mindfulness, including:

1. *Clutter-Free Environment*: A clean and organized space provides a sense of order and calmness. Clutter causes visual disturbances, requiring the brain to filter out additional distractions, overstimulating the mind, and decreasing concentration. To achieve a clutter-free environment, continuously check in with the space. "Does this item serve me daily?" If it does not, consider placing it in storage or simply out of your daily flow.
2. *Personalization and Comfort*: Grounding items serve to remind you of joy, family/friends, and sense of self. They offer comfort and emotional support. Taking the time to offer a sense of yourself brings pride to the space and will make it feel more at home. Examples include pictures of family/friends, seashells, art. There is, of course, a balance with clutter and grounding items. Check in with personal items to see if they still serve you as well.
3. *Functional Design*: Consider the functionality of your space. A well-designed and organized environment can enhance efficiency and productivity. When everything has a designated place and serves a purpose, it reduces the mental load associated with searching for items or navigating a cluttered space. Micro-inconvenience can add to the larger stress load. Try out different designs of a workspace so it services you. Perhaps move a printer to a more convenient location, and change the position of a desk so it is closer to the door.
4. *Optimize Lighting Exposure*:

   - During Night Shifts: Use bright, natural light or light therapy lamps to stay alert during the night. Exposure to bright light can help signal to your body that it's time to be awake.
   - After Night Shifts: Minimize exposure to bright light on your way home from work to signal to your body that it is time to wind down and prepare for sleep.

5. *Sensory Considerations*: Pay attention to the sensory aspects of your environment. Pleasant scents, comfortable textures, and soothing sounds can contribute to a more mindful and relaxing atmosphere. Consider incorporating elements like scented candles, soft blankets, or ambient music to enhance your space. Fresh flowers, eucalyptus, or elements of nature can bring life and positive sensory stimulation.
6. *Dedicated Mindfulness Areas*: Designate specific areas within your space for mindfulness activities such as meditation, yoga, or simply quiet reflection. Creating a designated space for these practices helps signal to your mind that it is time for relaxation and self-care.

Reflection Questions

- Is my space intentional?
- Can it make us more efficient?
- How do I use my space daily?

Part 2: Examples of Mindful Practices

Stretches for Surgeons on the Go

Our daily routines often place us in positions of flexion and force, whether it is holding laparoscopic instruments, typing extensively, or sitting for prolonged periods with our hips flexed in a chair. A fundamental approach to stretching involves countering the repetitive actions we engage in. For instance, after grasping laparoscopic tools for hours, consider incorporating stretches that involve hyperextending your fingers during a walk to your car, in the elevator, while you wait for your coffee! Bringing intention to the body parts we chronically use can improve daily practice as physicians and prevent long-term health complications.

Remember to breathe deeply and consistently during these stretches and never push yourself to the point of pain. Stretching should feel comfortable and help release tension in your body. Stretches can be held for as long or as little as you like.

Fingers	Open and close your hands as wide as they can go Hyperextend each finger Cross hands and turn inside out Massage base of metatarsals in small circles
Wrist	Place hands on table/floor, point fingers towards you Roll wrist, clockwise, then counter-clockwise
Shoulder	Fold hands together and flex them inside out in front of you. Rise to the sky. Place hand on wall and extend arm backwards Roll shoulders clockwise, then counter-clockwise
Side body	Raise hands to the sky, hold your right wrist with your left hand, and stretch left. Repeat on opposite side. Keep your spine long, twist your torso to the right. Repeat on opposite side.
Neck	Slowly tilt your head to one side, bringing your ear towards your shoulder. Repeat on opposite side. Turn your head to one side, looking over your shoulder. Repeat on the opposite side. Gently lower your chin towards your chest, feeling the stretch in the back of your neck.
Low Back and Hip Flexors	Let your arms hang down or reach for your shins or the floor. Stand with 1 foot forward and the other foot back. Bend your front knee and keep your back leg straight. Repeat on opposite side. While in a seated position, cross your right ankle over your left knee. Apply gentle pressure down on your right knee. Repeat on opposite side.
Calf and ankles	Stand about 1–2 feet away from a wall. Step your right foot forward and place the ball of that foot against the wall. Repeat on opposite side. Dorsiflex and plantarflex foot. Rotate in circle.

Just Breathe

Mindful breathing is the act of taking deliberate breaths to slow the nervous system and bring focus back into the present moment. Breathing exercises are a critical tool to use before, after, and during stressful encounters. These exercises can be carried out in just 10 seconds or longer as needed. Whether at a desk, before entering a patient room, or in response to unexpected challenges throughout the day, these exercises provide a valuable resource. In situations where frustration might trigger a reactive response, taking a deliberate breath can disrupt the cycle of stress and frustration imposed upon you.

Here's a simple mindful breathing exercise you can try:

- Find a quiet and comfortable place to sit or lie down.
- Close your eyes and bring your attention to your breath.
- Inhale slowly and deeply through your nose, counting to four.
- Exhale slowly and completely through your mouth, counting to six.
- Continue this pattern, focusing on the sensations of each breath.
- If your mind wanders, gently bring it back to your breath without judgment.

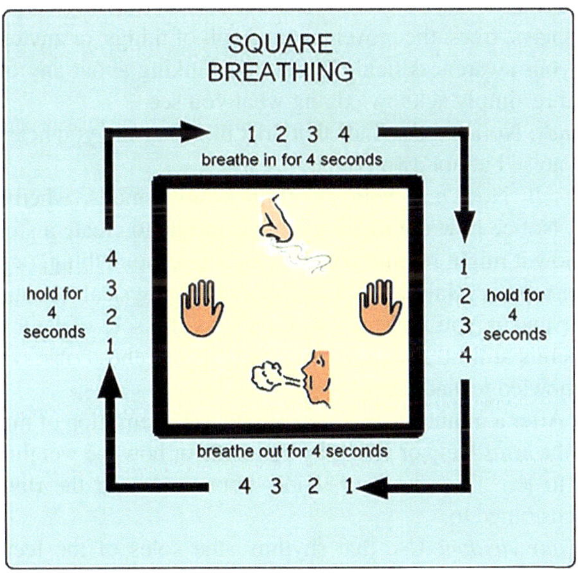

Source: Square Breathing For Kids—DEKIDRA. https://surreyschoolsone.ca/parents/all-learning-ideas/square-breathing

Meditation: Meditation While Walking and Working

Meditation like exercise takes practice and dedication. Doctors' minds often race with questions like "Did I choose the right treatment?" "How could I have done anything better during that surgery?" These questions often make it difficult to fall asleep at night. The goal of meditation is not to completely eliminate these thoughts but rather become an observer of them. Practicing meditation can be done at any moment you set an intention to do so. When walking from your car to the office, consider a trial of a walk meditation, rather than scrolling through patient charts or Instagram.

Headspace offers instructions on how to walk while meditating. Simply follow each cue for about 30–60 seconds:

1. *Body check*: As you start to walk, notice how the body feels. Heavy or light, stiff or relaxed? Take a few seconds to become aware of your posture and the way you're carrying yourself.
2. *Observe*: Without trying to change the way you're walking, simply observe your gait. Bring your attention to it. This can sometimes make you feel self-conscious, but that feeling usually passes.
3. *Tune in*: Tune into what's going on around you—passing cars, other people, window displays, trees, the movement and still of things, or any other sights that come into your awareness field. You're not thinking about any of these things, though; you're simply acknowledging what you see.
4. *Noting sounds*: Notice the sounds that drift in. What can you hear? Again, try to realize any noise but not dwell on it.
5. *Familiar smell*: Now turn your attention to any smells, whether pleasant or unpleasant. Notice how the mind habitually wants to create a story out of each smell and how it might remind you of somewhere, something, or someone.
6. *Physical sensations*: Make a point of noticing any physical sensations, from how the weather makes you feel to how it feels as the sole of your feet touch the ground. There's still no need to think about any of these observations. Simply notice, acknowledge, and let go.
7. *Movement*: After a minute or two, contemplate the sensation of movement in the body: how the arms hang or swing by your side or how the weight steadily shifts from right to left. Observe your stride, your pace, and the rhythm you have become accustomed to.
8. *Focus on your rhythm*: Use that rhythm—the soles of the feet touching the ground—as your base of awareness, a place you can mentally come back to when the mind wanders off. Repeat this throughout your walk, step by step, block by block, or mile by mile.

Mindful Journaling Practice

After a long day of work, physicians often compartmentalize their emotions and feelings without processing the events that they have been through. Journaling is a therapeutic way to bring light to our thoughts, feelings, and perceptions of daily events that are present in our subconscious. Journaling provides us with the opportunity to slow down from our busy schedules, reflect on our lives, and allow us to bring awareness into our surroundings and make changes if deemed necessary. Journaling is inexpensive and can be done on a computer, cell-phone, or pen and paper. Additionally, journaling does not have to solely be in the form of writing; it can be done through doodling, sketches, or other art forms. There is no correct way to journal; it should serve as a therapeutic outlet from a high stress demanding career.

Conclusion

Being an OBGYN is inherently high stress, placing significant demands on both physical and emotional well-being, often compounded by limited control over acute emergencies, working hours, and workload. However, amidst this chaos, we can retain agency over our response. Mindfulness, the capacity to cope and remain present, empowers us to regulate the extent to which external pressures affect our internal state. By observing a racing or intrusive thought, understanding the effect of the thought, and then ultimately separating self from negative thoughts provides capacity to enjoy the present moment and disrupt the detrimental impact of chronic stress on the body. Mindfulness is an individualized practice that is continuously growing and changing. Experimenting with different practices can help identify what works best for each person. Mindfulness interventions have shown to provide positive physical and psychological health outcomes which ultimately can decrease physician burnout and lead to increased work productivity and better patient outcomes.

References

1. Paturel A. When physicians are traumatized [Internet]. 13 Aug 2019 [cited 2024 May 7]. Available from: https://www.aamc.org/news/when-physicians-are-traumatized#:~.
2. Good DJ, Lyddy CJ, Glomb TM, Bono JE, Brown KW, Duffy MK, et al. Contemplating mindfulness at work. J Manag. 2015;42(1):114–42. https://doi.org/10.1177/0149206315617003.
3. Sevinc G, Hölzel BK, Hashmi J, Greenberg J, McCallister A, Treadway M, et al. Common and dissociable neural activity after mindfulness-based stress reduction and relaxation response

programs [Internet]. U.S. National Library of Medicine; 2018 [cited 2024 May 7]. Available from: https://www.ncbi.nlm.nih.gov/pmc/articles/PMC5976535/.

4. Greenberg J, Romero VL, Elkin-Frankston S, Bezdek MA, Schumacher EH, Lazar SW. Reduced interference in working memory following mindfulness training is associated with increases in hippocampal volume. Brain Imaging Behav. 2018;13(2):366–76. https://doi.org/10.1007/s11682-018-9858-4.
5. Waxenbaum JA. Anatomy, autonomic nervous system [Internet]. U.S. National Library of Medicine; 2023 [cited 2024 May 7]. Available from: https://www.ncbi.nlm.nih.gov/books/NBK539845/.
6. Gibson J. Mindfulness, interoception, and the body: a contemporary perspective [Internet]. U.S. National Library of Medicine; 2019 [cited 2024 May 7]. Available from: https://www.ncbi.nlm.nih.gov/pmc/articles/PMC6753170/.

Chapter 53
Developing and Maintaining Interests Outside of Medicine

Meredith Crisp Duffy

Similar to growing a practice, fostering interests outside of medicine takes a conscious effort. I never cared for the term work-life balance. I envisioned a balance scale, similar to the scales of justice. I knew that if laid on the scales, my work and life would not equate. I saw my life outside of medicine as the kindergartner on a teeter totter with a professional linebacker; my non-work life was looking down with no hopes of its feet ever touching the ground. To avoid being somewhat overwhelmed and dismayed by the concept, I put those thoughts aside and lived life. Luckily, over time, I learned that there is a way to enjoy all aspects of life and, instead of balance, I have found what I understand is work-life harmony. Work-life harmony describes a way in which individuals can blend their professional and personal lives together. In a Forbes article, Dr. Patti Fletcher suggests that one can achieve harmony by delegating when necessary, working as a team with mentors you trust and members you can mentor, and also allowing oneself time to rejuvenate [1].

Studies on the Blue Zones, areas throughout the world where people live 100 years of age at a much higher frequency, have provided insight into what appears to lead to a long, healthy life. Characteristics common to these centenarians are perceiving one's purpose, belonging to a spiritual group, placing one's loved ones as high priority, discarding stress, performing activities or chores that require movement throughout the day, and nutrition such as eating a plant-based diet and use of alcohol and food in moderation [2]. Similarly, to avoid burnout as a physician, it is important to "promote personal and professional well-being on all levels:

M. C. Duffy (✉)
Division of Gynecologic Oncology, MD Anderson Cancer Center at Cooper, Cooper Medical School of Rowan University and Cooper University Health Care, Camden, NJ, USA

A. Malik et al. (eds.), *An Obstetrician/Gynecologist's Path*,
https://doi.org/10.1007/978-3-031-87098-9_53

personal, emotional, psychological, and spiritual." Nurturing these areas in life should start during training and continue through one's career [3].

Not only is self-care important for the physician individually, but also for the care of his/her patients. Physician stress and burnout has been connected with provider-reported inferior quality of patient care [4, 5].

Most physicians already have some areas of interest. The Blue Zone research can serve as a useful guide to develop a balanced and harmonious life. The concept of work-life harmony suggests that your outside interests will only enhance your practice. For example, exercise can assist as a stress relief and prepare your body for a day in the operating room. A spiritual connection may be grounding when breaking bad news or traversing the obstacles of medical practice or a pandemic. A healthy diet can assist with health goals and potentially lead to a longer, healthier life for all passions, professional and personal. Personal relationships can help you relate to your patients in an authentic way.

There can be constraints to developing outside interests. One constraint is time, both during training and once in practice. First, time spent at work can be long during training and in early practice. Work hours are no longer monitored after entering practice, and it can be difficult to scale back the hours with which one has become accustomed. Establishing oneself as a new provider, growing a practice, and meeting ongoing education requirements all require a regular time commitment. In order to leave time for necessary work obligations, it is helpful to develop a routine schedule for the day or week to allot time to professional and personal interests.

Another time challenge can be the demands of spouse, children, parents, and friends. These demands can either be self-imposed by one's personal expectations or by the pressure of others. To tackle your outside interests, you will also need to set boundaries with work and friends. I suggest you designate time while still at work to complete electronic medical records, answer work emails, and work on research. Dedicate time as well to things you enjoy outside of work and put work-related tasks aside. A good habit is to answer non-urgent work emails during designated hours. If you answer non-urgent emails and texts at 2 am or while on vacation, you are setting a tone that you are always available and your personal time is not valuable. Not only are you setting a tone for those who work with you, but also for yourself and your family. It can be a hard expectation to break if healthy boundaries are not set early on. I often hear that providers plan to check off the items on their bucket list when they retire. As we learn during a medical career, we are not guaranteed tomorrow, much less retirement. Seize the day. Cross off some of those dreams now, while your health is good, and then start adding more dreams to your bucket list. Take time on your days off and use your vacation time. Consider it valuable time to reconnect with your family, friends, and yourself. Time to rejuvenate is important.

Another obstacle to maintaining outside interests is finances. If a hobby is expensive, extra work may be required to pay for the boat, club membership, or international travel. If one's house payment is so high that it is hard to make ends meet on a set salary, this can cause stress and create a need to constantly push to work more. My intention is not to suggest you find a cheaper hobby but perhaps consider your overall expenses. If your hobby, house, and car are all expensive, the harmony of life may be flat. During my medical school orientation, someone from the finance department explained "if you live like a doctor when you are a medical student, you will live like a medical student when you are a doctor." You are likely past those medical school days if you are reading this, but I feel sentiment holds true throughout a career. Living within or beneath your means can reduce the stresses which come when living paycheck to paycheck. If you are not encumbered by multiple, pricy bills, you give yourself more freedom to enjoy life outside of medicine and shed some stress.

Another financial topic of importance is retirement. Hard to believe you should start thinking of retirement when you are completing your training and just starting practice, but there is no time like the present. Not only do you want to develop outside interests to maintain harmony during your career, but you are developing passions you can enjoy through retirement. Many friends from a variety of professions struggle with the first few months of retirement and later tell me they don't know how they had time to work. They now fill their days with the things they have always loved, including volunteering, hobbies, and family. Most of these passions were developed prior to retirement, but retirement allows more time to enjoy them. To assist in financial planning, I highly recommend you find a qualified financial planner who can guide you on how to pay off student loans and how to budget and plan for your future. Lastly, regarding finances, I would encourage you to sign up for specialty-specific disability insurance. This is an investment, but it can give peace of mind if an accident or long-term illness prevents you from practicing and generating an income.

Residency and early career are an exciting time. You have worked hard to achieve goals of getting into school, matching into residency and then landing that first job. Consciously setting boundaries and planning will allow you to find a healthy harmony in life which will aid in satisfaction with your career and overall life.

References

1. Fletcher P. Work-life balance is over: let's talk about work-life harmony. Forbes. https://www.forbes.com/sites/forbeshumanresourcescouncil/2020/11/13/work-life-balance-is-over-lets-talk-about-work-life-harmony/?sh=7f293e825b48. 13 Nov 2020.
2. Buettner D, Skemp S. Blue zones: lessons from the world's longest lived. Am J Lifestyle Med. 2016;10:318–21.
3. Spickard A, Gabbe S, Christensen J. Mid-career burnout in generalist and specialist physicians. JAMA. 2002;288:1447–50.
4. Shanafelt T, et al. Burnout and self-reported patient care in an internal medicine residency program. Ann Intern Med. 2002;136:358–67.
5. Firth-Cozens J, et al. Doctors' perceptions of links between stress and lowered clinical care. Soc Sci Med. 1997;44:1017–22.

Index

A. Malik et al. (eds.), *An Obstetrician/Gynecologist's Path*,
https://doi.org/10.1007/978-3-031-87098-9

GPSR Compliance

The European Union's (EU) General Product Safety Regulation (GPSR) is a set of rules that requires consumer products to be safe and our obligations to ensure this.

If you have any concerns about our products, you can contact us on ProductSafety@springernature.com

In case Publisher is established outside the EU, the EU authorized representative is:

Springer Nature Customer Service Center GmbH
Europaplatz 3
69115 Heidelberg, Germany

Batch number: 10732632

Printed by Printforce, the Netherlands